THE
COLOUR
FIT
METHOD

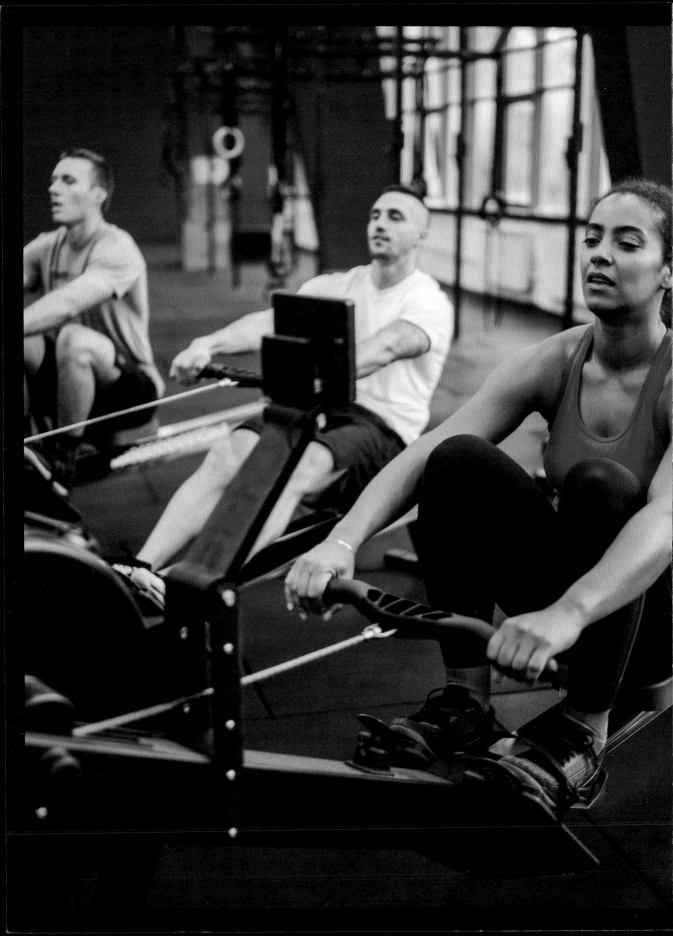

The secret nutrition
and fitness plan used
by elite athletes

THE
COLOUR
FIT
METHOD

Transform your body shape,
energy and health

DR TOM LITTLE

PIATKUS

Dedicated to my mum, Jennifer Little – the bravest woman I know

PIATKUS
First published in Great Britain in 2022 by Piatkus
1 3 5 7 9 10 8 6 4 2

A CIP catalogue record for this book is available from the British Library.

ISBN 978-0-349-42878-9

Book design: D.R. ink
Food photography: Ian Garlick
Food styling: Lorna Brash
Illustrations: Emil Dacanay
General photography: p.2 martin-dm, Getty Images; p.3 Chris Parkes; p.9 Gorodenkoff, Adobe Stock; p.12 Thomas Barwick, Getty Images; p.200 nastasic, Getty Images; p.224 lacaosa, Getty Images; p257 Solskin, Getty Images; p273 Malcolm Couzens, Getty Images.

Printed and bound in Italy by L.E.G.O. S.p.A.
Papers used by Piatkus are from well-managed forests and other responsible sources.

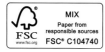

FSC
www.fsc.org
MIX
Paper from responsible sources
FSC® C104740

Piatkus
An imprint of
Little, Brown Book Group
Carmelite House
50 Victoria Embankment
London EC4Y 0DZ

An Hachette UK Company
www.hachette.co.uk
www.littlebrown.co.uk

Disclaimer
The dietary information and exercises in this book are not intended to replace or conflict with the advice given to you by your GP or other health professionals. All matters regarding your health should be discussed with your GP. The author and publisher disclaim any liability directly or indirectly from the use of the material in this book by any person.

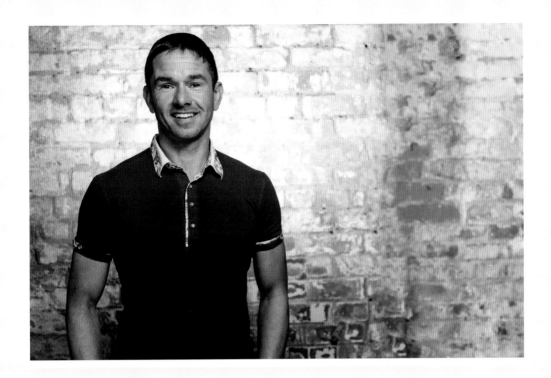

About the author

Dr Tom Little is a performance and nutrition specialist with over twenty years' experience in professional sport and fitness. He has worked primarily at football clubs in the Premier League and Championship, including Manchester City, Burnley, Leeds United, Nottingham Forest and Sheffield Wednesday. A finalist for the 'Fabrice Muamba Award for Outstanding Services to Football Medicine and Science', he has consulted for the English and New Zealand FA, Nike, and combat, tennis and rugby sport athletes, in addition to a wide spectrum of amateur athletes. Tom has a BSc, MSc & PhD in Sports Science and Nutrition, has published several peer-reviewed papers and is a regular speaker at conferences. He is a registered sport and exercise nutritionist (SENR) and an accredited strength and conditioning coach (ASCC).

Tom founded Colour-Fit in 2016 and merged with wellbeing company hero in 2018, to rebrand as heroPro, and provide a leading nutritional and fitness app. Customers have included Manchester City, Chelsea, Manchester United, Arsenal, Leicester City, Brighton, WRU and Lion's Rugby, Melbourne Demons, Saracens, Leicester Tigers, FC Copenhagen, DC United and British Judo. For more information visit www.heroprosport.com.

Tom is currently Head of Performance at Preston North End. He is a keen amateur athlete and has won several adventure races, including the infamous Tough Guy. He lives in the Peak District with his wife Emma and two children – Isabelle and James.

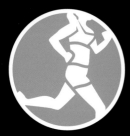 **PERFORMANCE FUEL**

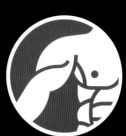 **LEAN MUSCLE**

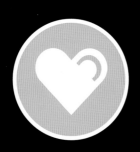 **HEALTH**

CONTENTS

Introduction

What is Colour-Fit?

The Colour-Fit Methodology is a revolutionary approach to nutrition and fitness that allows you to easily achieve your health, fitness and appearance ambitions. Conceived within elite sport, the Colour-Fit Methodology has benefited countless top-flight athletes all around the globe, but the principles of Colour-Fit apply to everyone, and this book represents the first time the methodology has been revealed to all.

Born of frustration

Like all the best inventions, Colour-Fit was born of frustration. If I had not invented the system, I would have probably murdered half of my players! I'd been a fitness and nutrition specialist working in elite sport for over two decades. I had a PhD and a string of other letters after my name, won awards and spoken at international conferences, and my work had been published in scientific journals. As an expert and keen amateur athlete, I have an unwavering belief in the benefits of good nutrition and training. If you could get the same benefits from a pill, everyone in the world would want to take it and benefit from enhanced energy, appearance, performance, mood, brain function, life span, libido, injury and disease resistance ... the list is endless.

Yet, season after season, I kept coming up against the same problem: despite all the work we did and the information I gave to players, they didn't seem to be able to put what I taught them about nutrition into practice. Fundamental principles – what to eat, when to eat it and how to make it – were somehow not getting through. I regularly saw players who, outwardly, looked in peak fitness but were actually underperforming, overweight and fundamentally unhealthy. As a coach who lives and dies by his players' prowess, I knew I had to do something.

There was one player, a talented young footballer who'd been recruited by a top club when he was eight years old, who ate tinned ravioli before a match. Afterwards, he'd head straight to Nando's to gorge on chicken wings. He had grasped a vague understanding of nutrition basics – carbs to fuel exercise, protein to repair muscle – but his interpretation of the 'rules' was too basic: carbs were simply pasta and bread; protein meant meat and protein powders. Like so many people, he didn't know how to choose and prepare healthy meals and was

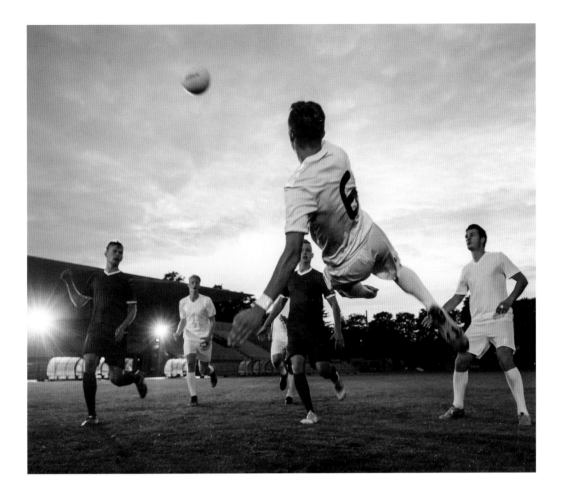

unsure of the constitution of the vast array of foods available and how they can help us to achieve our goals. As a result, he ate out frequently, consumed lots of processed foods and avoided whole foods – the ones that are loaded with carbs *and* proteins plus a whole load of essential vitamins and minerals. As a result, his health was compromised and his performance was inconsistent.

Footballers aren't necessarily renowned for their smarts, but I knew this wasn't simply a matter of brawn over brains. If they are lucky enough to sign pro contracts, many young players are plunged into the real world where they are expected to fend for themselves. Unfortunately, most don't have the know-how or confidence to cook meals, and although there are lots of recipes out there, to a cooking novice they can appear complex and intimidating. But good nutritious food can be simple to prepare *and* taste amazing.

Social media certainly doesn't help either. I have seen countless athletes follow fitness gurus who dole out conflicting, impractical information without backing any of it up with actual science, leaving their followers ill-informed and bamboozled.

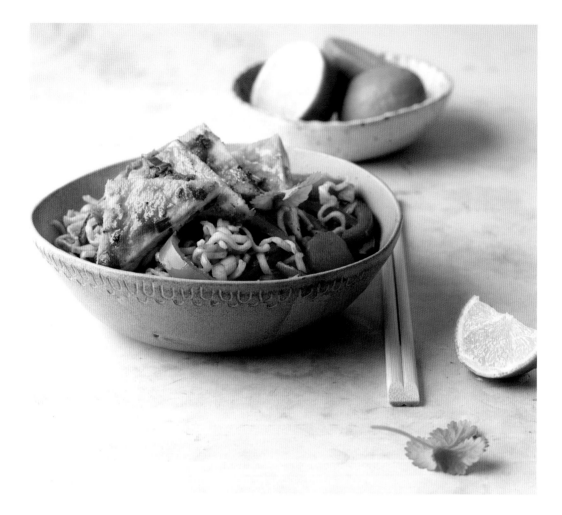

If this sounds like you or someone you know, it's because people everywhere – not only footballers and athletes, but anyone who eats food and moves their body – are facing the same fundamental issues: complex, impractical, rigid and unfounded advice that all too often brings poor results.

Eureka! It ain't what you say, it's the way that you say it

I tried everything to get the right messages across: I designed posters for the changing rooms, gave talks and cookery demonstrations. I even went shopping with clients to help them buy the right foods. But while the odd head of broccoli might occasionally show up in someone's fridge, nothing really changed. Why wasn't the message getting through?

The lightbulb moment came one evening as I was working at the kitchen table. My son, then six years old, was messing about on my phone. I noticed how he seemed to know instinctively how everything worked. The design on the phone guided his choices and made it easy for him to navigate to where he wanted to go. *Ding!* What if I could design an intuitive way to help people achieve their fitness and health goals? Now that *was* a tasty idea! With my son climbing over me, I played around with a few ideas for how it could look. Within moments he pointed and said, 'that one makes you run' and 'that one makes you healthy'. I'd cracked it with a six-year-old; I might just have a chance with food-prep-phobic athletes.

Since those humble beginnings in my kitchen, Colour-Fit has taken professional sport by storm. Thousands of elite sports teams and athletes now use the Colour-Fit system through the hero navigator app – from premiership football and rugby championship teams to golfers and world-champion combat and motor-sports athletes. It's a foolproof, secret system that ensures that elite athletes achieve their goals. Except, here's the thing, it's not a secret system and it's not only for elite athletes – it's for everyone!

Shared goals and barriers

We might worship elite athletes, but they have the same goals and problems as you and me. We all share goals that involve being healthy, changing our body shape and/or maximising our performance. Athletes might be more focused on performance, whether fuelling for a big race, losing weight for a mountain stage or bulking up to be stronger in the tackle, but many of us weekend warriors share similar ambitions. If you're not an athlete you might think that you haven't got a goal, but you probably still have one or two. If all you want to do is stay exactly as you are, that's a goal. Whether it's short term or long term, a big impact or a tiny tweak, to lose a few pounds, improve your health, train for a marathon or just walk the dog without getting out of breath, these are all goals that Colour-Fit can help you reach for. And because everyone's goals and activity levels can change day by day, Colour-Fit flexes to work with you at every stage of your journey.

Athletes also face the same barriers that we do in achieving their goals. We all need help making suitable choices as to how we train and eat, and we need the knowledge and confidence to carry out these choices. The Colour-Fit Methodology uses colours, names and icons that allow you to select suitable meals and training methods instinctively to achieve your goals. I empower you to carry out your choices by making the meals and training as simple and practical as possible. Throughout the book I explain the rationales behind the Colour-Fit system so that you can easily understand and adapt the methodology to suit your unique lifestyle and circumstances.

As for the secret, I'm happy to admit there's nothing new about the theories underpinning Colour-Fit (but don't tell anyone). Everything is based on the latest peer-reviewed, evidence-based science. In this sense I haven't invented a new system, I've simply gathered information from the world's brightest and best in the fields of training and nutrition to bring it all together in a way that everyone can not only understand but also live by.

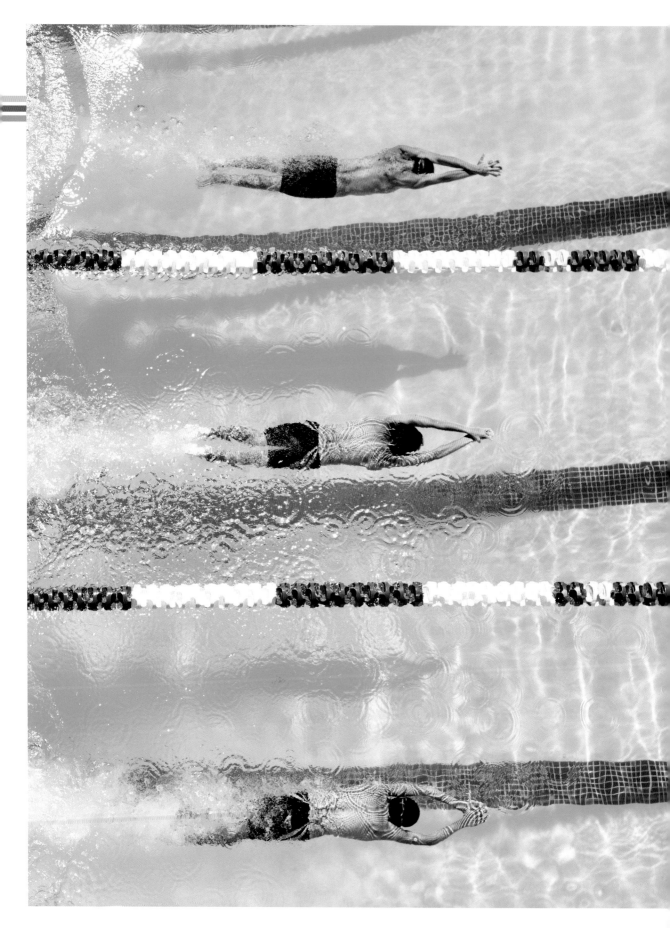

Colour-Fit Cook, Colour-Fit Train and Colour-Fit Plans

My aim in this book is to give you all the tools you will need to achieve your fitness, health and appearance goals. I start with Colour-Fit Cook, which contains over 120 delicious, easy-to-make meals, each with my unique Colour-Fit plate system to help you intuitively choose appropriate meals, and links to video demonstrations to give you confidence and the know-how to make the meal. I also provide my favourite meal builders, which enable you to design an endless variety of meals to suit your goals. Next, Colour-Fit Training describes the training methods used in the book and how I have adapted training to make it simpler to understand and carry out. Finally, Colour-Fit Plans bring everything together to provide training and nutrition plans for various fitness, sport and body-shape goals. The plans are not only highly effective but easy to understand and carry out (with a bit of willpower), thanks to the Colour-Fit Training Load Gauges and links to video demonstrations.

So now it's your turn

The young lad who ate ravioli from tins and loved his Nando's is now a well-known elite football player. Of course, I can't put it all down to Colour-Fit, but it certainly made him leaner and improved his energy, mood and health. As a result, we saw his match performance rocket. Result!

I've seen the same transformation take place time and again with every athlete who I let in on the Colour-Fit secret. And I've heard the same thing from world champions through to Joe Bloggs: Colour-Fit works because it's so simple and practical, which means you can stick at it long term.

Now you know the secret of some of the world's top athletes, it's your turn to pick it up and run with it. Remember, this isn't a rigid diet plan; you can do this and see amazing results, whether you're an Olympic swimmer or a champion couch potato. I'm made up to be sharing Colour-Fit with you at last and helping you live a more colourful life. I can't wait for you to experience the simple pleasure of achieving your goals, whatever they may be.

Ready? Get set, go!

Dr Tom Little

PART 1
COLOUR-FIT COOK

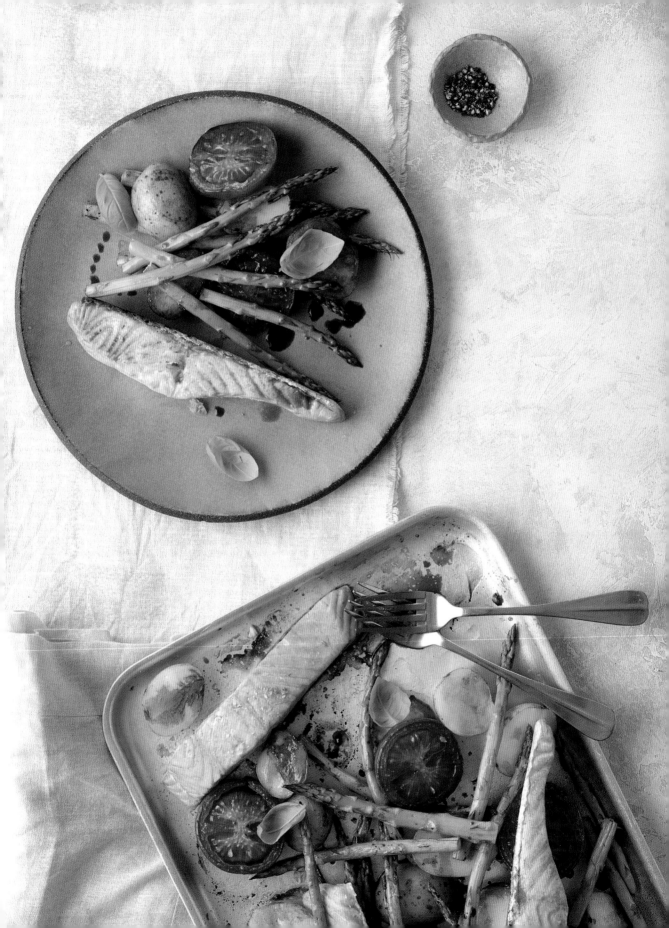

In Colour-Fit Cook you will find a vast array of delicious, easy-to-make meals that have been specifically designed to have a proven benefit for health or fitness. More than this, Colour-Fit Cook revolutionises our approach to food via the Colour-Fit plates associated with each meal. With just a quick glance, the Colour-Fit plate intuitively gives you all the information you need about whether a meal is suitable for achieving your nutrition and fitness goals.

How Colour-Fit works

Using Colour-Fit is as easy as 1, 2, 3:

1 Identify your goal

Colour-Fit works by dividing your goals into three core categories. At any time, most of us are working towards at least one of these goals, if not all three:

1. Increased performance (train harder, perform better, lead a more active lifestyle)
2. Desired body shape (achieving the body shape we want: slimming down, toning or bulking up)
3. Improved health (improved energy, mood, immunity, appearance and sleep)

2 Match your goal to the Colour-Fit colours

Once you've identified your goal, you can match it to the three core Colour-Fit goals, each represented by an intuitive name, colour and icon.

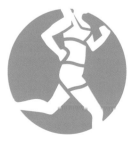

Performance fuel

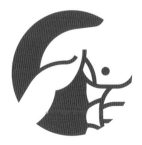

Lean muscle

Health

The three icons

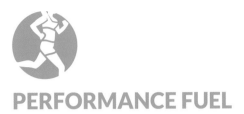

PERFORMANCE FUEL

To maximise exercise performance
(running icon, colour – green for go)

Performance Fuel represents net carbohydrates (carbs), which are found in foods such as wholegrains, fruit and vegetables. They are the body's most efficient *fuel* source and they therefore maximise *performance* when we need to smash it on the pitch or in the gym, or to support an active lifestyle. Net carbs are total carbs minus fibre, which represents the carbs we can absorb to use for fuel. Carbs are an important fuel source for many of our bodily functions and our brain's preferred source of energy. If carbs are low, our maximum exercise capacity is reduced, coordination and concentration are impaired and we are more at risk of infection and injury. One of the core principles of Colour-Fit is that we vary the proportion of Performance Fuel foods in line with our activity levels and exercise demands, a process known as 'carb periodisation'. When you are training hard, look for a higher proprtion of green in your Colour-Fit plates, to support performance. If you are not active, lessen the amount of fuel foods so you can prioritise health and/or body-shape goals instead. Also, energy requirements will be less, so reducing fuel will help avoid a potential excess energy intake, which would lead to weight gain over time.

An exception would be low-carb or fasted training, where you deliberately train when you have low carb stores. This can promote the use of fat for energy and enhance aerobic enymes (these help create energy) when you only want to train moderately. Remember, though, your performance potential, and therefore performance improvements, will be greater when you have higher carb stores.

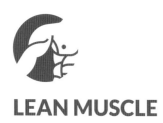

LEAN MUSCLE

For desired body shape and repair
(six-pack icon, colour – red for a metabolism that is fired up)

Lean Muscle represents proteins. Proteins, which are found in foods such as meat, fish, eggs and soya products, are critical in our diet, as they form the building blocks for all our cells. They are excellent for staying *lean* or losing weight for several reasons. Because of their critical function, sufficient protein intake is closely regulated by our appetite. As such, proteins fill us up for longer compared to carbs and fats, as they slow stomach emptying and stimulate the release of appetite-regulating hormones in the gut. Proteins also have the lowest net calories: proteins and carbs contain 4 kcal per gram, and fat 9 kcal, but protein requires the most energy to digest and absorb. Proteins are also the building blocks of *muscle*, which has a high metabolic rate, helping us to burn more energy 24/7. In combination with strength training, protein promotes muscle tone and definition and, following strenuous exercise, protein helps to quickly repair and build muscle.

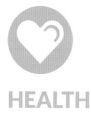

HEALTH

For improved health
(heart icon, colour – gold for a healthy glow)

Nutrients from our food are key to our well-being, energy levels, mood and appearance. As such, they are non-negotiable, and play a part in every Colour-Fit meal. To measure health, I invented the health score, which asseses quantities of vitamins, minerals, fibre and healthy fats that are essential to our health, and added sugar and saturated fat that are generally poor for our health. The higher the score, the healthier the meal. A health score of 5 would indicate that you are getting five of your daily recommended intakes of vitamins, minerals, fibre or omega-3 fats, akin to getting your five-a-day. You can prioritise those meals with a high Health proportion if you aren't doing anything unusual on the exercise front and just want to stay healthy, feel good and maintain a healthy weight. Colour-Fit recipes also provide a nutritional breakdown for each meal, and indicate if a meal is high in a specific health element.

Calories are king

Calories are also key to body shape, fitness and health goals, so look for the calorie load indicator on the outside of each Colour-Fit plate. Like a speed dial, this is a quick, at-a-glance way to stay on top of your calories, with a full dial representing 900 calories. In general, look for: higher calorie loads if you have increased activity/exercise demands or if you want to gain muscle; mid-range if you are moderately active; and moderate-to-lower calorie loads if you want to lose weight.

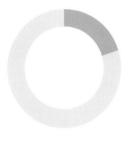

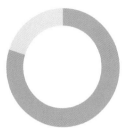

Low calorie load   **High calorie load**

3 Plate up!

Use the Colour-Fit plate symbol next to each recipe to see instantly if a meal is right for you and your goals. Some examples:

(a) Are you training hard or looking to maximise exercise performance? Look for a high proportion of Performance Fuel foods on your Colour-Fit plates with moderate-to-higher calorie loads (below left). If you are exercising moderately and exercise performance isn't that important, look for a fairly balanced Colour-Fit plate (below right).

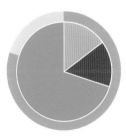

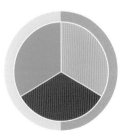

Performance for hard exercise   **Performance for moderate exercise**
High Performance Fuel   Moderate Performance Fuel
and calorie load   and calorie load

(b) Do you want to stay lean or are you aiming to lose weight? Look for more Lean Muscle foods and lower-to-moderate calorie loads. Generally, look for meals and foods high in Health, as it is important for our metabolism and ensures that we are nutritionally fulfilled, which reduces hunger. Vary Performance Fuel in line with your activity levels, but generally aim to keep it quite low to reduce insulin levels and thereby promote fat burning. High-carb diets can certainly produce weight loss, as long as calories are kept in check, but a high protein intake has been proven to be optimal for long-term weight loss.

(c) Perhaps you have just killed it in a HIIT session and need to promote recovery or build muscle. Prioritise plates that are higher in Lean Muscle, to repair and build muscle, and Performance Fuel to restore energy and promote nutrient uptake via insulin. Calorie loads should be moderate to high.

(d) Have you been burning the candle at both ends or want to boost your immune system? You can prioritise Health foods on your plate if you want to improve your general health, feel good and maintain a healthy weight, especially if you are not too fussed about exercise performance.

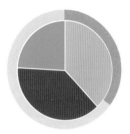

Weight loss
High Lean Muscle and Health, low-to-moderate Performance Fuel and calorie load

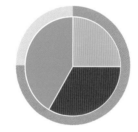

Recovery from hard exercise or building muscle
High Fuel, Lean Muscle and calorie load

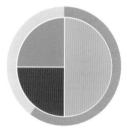

Maximising health
High Health, moderate calories

For many people who are moderately active and happy with their body shape and health, having a fairly even overall Colour-Fit plate is fine. However, if you want to maximise performance levels, change weight or really improve your health, more targeted nutrition is optimal. But, don't worry, you'll soon find that Colour-Fit plates are intuitive, simple and fast; there is no need to resolutely track calories or macros. Simply be guided by the colours on your Colour-Fit plates to reach your goals.

Despite the benefits of targeted nutrition, please don't become obsessed with every meal. Food should be one of life's joys and not something to stress over. The key to successful long-term nutrition is to be in the right ballpark *most* of the time. This 'flexible' eating pattern has been shown to be more successful than following a rigid dietary regime.

If you have a keen interest in nutrition and want more detailed nutritional information, you can head to hero navigator, MyFitnessPal or FatSecret, where you can find the Colour-Fit meals.

Recipes for success

All Colour-Fit recipes have been designed by my expert team, whose mission it is to combine optimal nutrition with a process that is practical and fuss-free. There are no lengthy lists of hard-to-find ingredients or bizarre machines required – this is real, unpretentious, practical food that, most importantly, tastes great! And, because Colour-Fit is for everyone, you'll find that there are plenty of vegetarian and vegan choices too (Colour-Fit is proud to be endorsed by FIFA's only recognised vegan sports club, Forest Green Rovers).

Kitchen know-how and having the confidence to give new recipes a go is a very real stumbling block for many people. Colour-Fit helps you to clear this hurdle by including step-by-step video demonstrations for every meal in the book. These can be accessed via the QR code on each meal page, using your phone or tablet. Note that the demonstrations are not designed to exactly follow the printed recipes but to be a useful addition for those who like visual guidance.

The recipes are divided into Breakfasts, Light Meals, Main Meals, Side Dishes, Snacks and Desserts, and Smoothies. Each meal has a Colour-Fit plate so that you'll know instantly if it is suitable for your goal.

Meet the meal builders

As an extra bonus, we also provide 'meal builders' at the end of each meal section. There are meals and snacks that I come back to again and again because they are so versatile, easy to make and because they pack a major nutritional punch: stir-fries, smoothies, salads, tray roasts, overnight oats and protein balls. Many of us know how to make these things, but it's easy to get stuck in a rut and find yourself making the same things on repeat. Meal builders show you the many options that you can choose from when putting together these popular recipes. This makes it easy for you to build meals that suit your goals and tastes; they also throw in some ideas as to how to switch up these simple super heroes – and they teach you cooking independence rather than just how to follow recipes.

The Colour-Fit Recipes

PERFORMANCE
FUEL

LEAN
MUSCLE

HEALTH

Light Meals

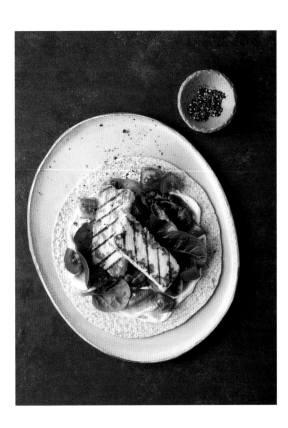

The Colour-Fit Recipes

PERFORMANCE FUEL
 LEAN MUSCLE
 HEALTH

 Healthy Chicken Pie (page 115)

 Rapid Chicken Sunday Dinner (page 116)

 Turkey Burgers with Feta and Spinach (page 118)

 Chill con Carne (page 119)

Meat

 Beef-Stuffed Peppers (page 120)

 Beef Stroganoff (page 121)

 Chinese Beef Noodles (page 123)

 Sweet Potato Cottage Pie (page 124)

 Lamb Kefta (page 125)

 Doner Kebab (page 126)

 Moussaka (page 128)

 Minute Steak with Roasted Peppers and Avocado Salad (page 129)

Stir-fry Meal Builder (page 130)

Tray Roast Meal Builder (page 132)

Side Dishes

 Spiced Bulgur Wheat (page 135)

 Cabbage Salad (page 136)

 Curried Cauli Rice (page 137)

 Tabbouleh (page 138)

 Cajun Street Rice (page 140)

 Loaded But Light Potato Skins (page 141)

 Pea, Watercress and Carrot Salad (page 143)

 Balsamic Kale (page 144)

 Leeks, Peas and Quinoa (page 145)

 Salt and Pepper Sweet Potato Chips (page 146)

The Colour-Fit Recipes

 Mushroom Bruschetta (page 148)

 Roasted Vegetables (page 149)

 Basil Pesto Gnocchi (page 151)

 Ratatouille (page 152)

 Sweet-and-Sour Crispy Asian Sprouts (page 153)

Snacks and Desserts

 Sushi Rolls (page 155)

 Lettuce and Tuna Boats (page 156)

 Courgette and Turkey Rolls (page 157)

 Almond Cobbler (page 157)

 Edamame Summer Rolls (page 158)

 Joint Jellies (page 160)

 Boiled Egg with Hummus and Cucumber (page 161)

 Almond and Berry Balls (page 163)

 Carrot Cake Balls (page 164)

 Mango and Coconut Balls (page 165)

 Apricot and Dark Chocolate Fuel Bars (page 166)

 Walnut Chocolate Truffles (page 168)

 Apple, Oat and Mixed Seed Bars (page 169)

 Avocado Brownies (page 171)

 Banana and Date Flapjacks (page 172)

 Fig, Hazelnut and Dark Chocolate Bars (page 173)

 Banana Bread (page 175)

 Blueberry and Banana Oat Muffins (page 176)

 Joint Panna Cotta (page 177)

 Healthy Eton Mess (page 178)

These recipes were designed to be used in tandem with the fitness plans in Part 3, but of course you can use them according to your own fitness needs – simply see the guidance on pages 19–21 on how to use the plate diagrams to meet your requirements. You'll also find some helpful information about preparing the recipes below.

NOTES ON THE RECIPES

- Vegetables, fruit, eggs, tortilla wraps, etc., are medium unless otherwise specified.
- Tablespoon and teaspoon measurements are level.
- Olive oil is suggested in the recipes, but you can also use rapeseed oil or coconut oil if you prefer. Do not use extra virgin olive oil for cooking; light olive oil is more suitable.
- Choose free-range eggs where possible.

You will see that some of the recipes are marked as gluten-free but please be aware that anyone who wishes to avoid *all* gluten will need to check products such as oats, stock cubes and ready-made sauces to ensure they buy gluten-free versions. Where recipes are vegan, or ingredients can be readily swapped for vegan alternatives, this is also indicated.

Many people like the convenience of using cup measures for ingredients that are easy to scoop or pour, so these are included for some dry ingredients, such as oats and flour.

BREAKFASTS

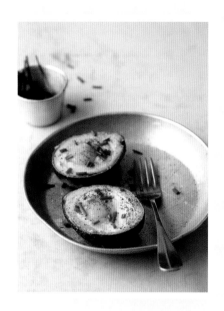

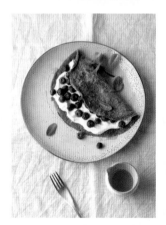

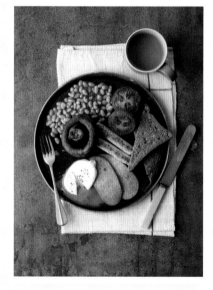

Apple and Cinnamon Pancakes

Serves 1

Prep. 8 minutes

Vegetarian, gluten-free

By using apples, oats and cinnamon you can make pancakes that taste great and are more healthy than the traditional recipe. As with most pancakes, they are fuel dominant, but they also provide some protein via the egg, milk and oats. Apples add a range of vitamins and fibre, and the eggs also provide vitamins, minerals and healthy fats. Cinnamon is a traditional warming spice to cook with apples, plus it has anti-inflammatory properties.

1 dessert apple, grated

2 tbsp low-fat natural yogurt

40g (scant ½ cup) porridge oats

50ml skimmed milk

¼ tsp ground cinnamon

1 tsp honey

2 eggs

2 tsp olive oil

1. Put 1 tbsp of the grated apple in a small bowl and add the yogurt. Mix well and set aside for the pancake topping.

2. Put the oats in a food processor or blender and add the remaining apple, the milk, cinnamon, honey and eggs. Blitz until smooth.

3. Heat a frying pan over a medium heat and add the oil.

4. Pour in the mixture to make small pancake shapes in the pan. Cook for 1–2 minutes until golden brown, then carefully flip and cook for a further 1–2 minutes. Transfer to a plate and keep warm. Repeat with the remaining mixture. Add the yogurt topping and serve.

Nutrition: Health score 2.4 High in iron, manganese and phosphorus

Kcal	Carbs	Sugar	Protein	Fat	Sat Fat	Fibre
198.5	26.7g	10.7g (11.9%)	8g	5.2g	4.1g (5.5%)	4.4g (14.7%)

Mango and Banana Parfait

Serves 1

Prep. 6 minutes

Vegetarian

½ mango or 85g frozen mango chunks

1 banana

50g sugar-free granola

4 tbsp Greek yogurt, or vegan alternative

This vitamin-C packed parfait is a refreshing way to set up your day. Bananas are a great fuel option containing lots of B vitamins and potassium to aid energy metabolism.

1. Using a sharp knife, score squares into the mango flesh and then push the skin side inwards to make the mango cubes stand proud. Cut off the cubes.

2. Put the banana, mango and 1 tbsp water in a food processor or blender and blitz to make a smooth paste.

3. Put the fruit purée in a glass and top with layers of granola and yogurt. Serve.

Nutrition: Health score 7.7 High in vitamins B1, A, C and folate

Kcal	Carbs	Sugar	Protein	Fat	Sat Fat	Fibre
402	77.4g	45.9g (51%)	12.8g	3.6g	1g (5.1%)	8.6g (22.5%)

Mocha Parfait

Serves 1

Prep. 3 minutes

20g (1 scoop) chocolate protein powder

1 tbsp cocoa powder

1 teaspoon instant coffee

6 tbsp low-fat Greek yogurt

2 tbsp granola

a small handful of blueberries

This is a great breakfast for all coffee lovers out there as it also provides a good amount of healthy protein.

1. Place the protein powder, cocoa, coffee and half the yogurt in a bowl and mix until smooth. Transfer the mixture into a glass jar or serving bowl.

2. Add a layer of the granola, then the rest of the yogurt and finally place the blueberries on top.

Nutrition: Health score 4.4. High in vitamins B2, B12 and calcium, manganese, phosphorus and selenium

Kcal	Carbs	Sugar	Protein	Fat	Sat Fat	Fibre
286.8	21.7g	13.9g (15.4%)	30.5g	7.8g	2.5g (12.6%)	3.6g (11.9%)

Apple and Date Bircher

Serves 1

Prep. 5 minutes

Vegan, gluten-free

This version of Bircher porridge follows the tradition by using apple juice, plus the fresh apple adds flavour and a great crunch. It has impressive health credentials with virtually the full spectrum of minerals. The chia seeds and walnuts add healthy fats and several minerals. This breakfast is principally carb-based so it's a good choice if you have an active day ahead.

150ml apple juice

1 dessert apple

50g (½ cup) porridge oats

8 pitted dried dates, chopped

4 tbsp Greek yogurt, or vegan alternative

1 tbsp chia seeds

a small handful of walnuts, crushed

1 tsp vanilla extract

1. Put all the ingredients in a bowl or a small sealable glass jar and mix well.

2. Leave in the fridge overnight or for a minimum of 20 minutes. Serve.

Nutrition: Health score 8.1 High in vitamins B2, K and magnesium

Kcal	Carbs	Sugar	Protein	Fat	Sat Fat	Fibre
747	123g	86g (96%)	18g	17g	1.7g (8.5%)	19g (51%)

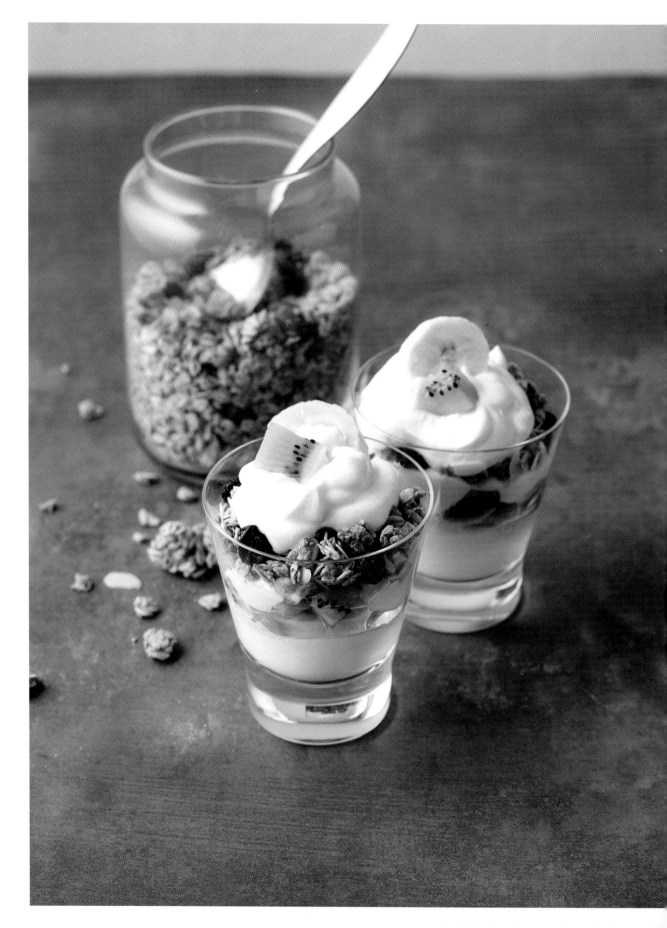

Kiwi and Banana Parfait

Serves 2

Prep. 8 minutes

Vegan

Yogurt, banana and tangy fresh kiwi combine for a zingy taste of the tropics. This versatile parfait can be used as a quick-fix breakfast or a mid-afternoon snack and is rich in protein, carbohydrate and vitamin C to help support recovery from training and minimise the risk of illness and infection.

3 tbsp Greek yogurt, or vegan alternative

1 tbsp honey or maple syrup

1 tsp vanilla extract

1 banana, sliced

1 kiwi, skinned and chopped

1 tbsp granola

1. Put the yogurt in a bowl and add the honey or maple syrup and vanilla. Mix together.

2. Spoon some of the mixture into two glasses. Put a layer of banana on top and then put some kiwi slices around the edge of each glass.

3. Spoon in some more yogurt mixture, and then the granola. Add some more yogurt, banana and kiwi, and serve.

Nutrition: Health score 4.9 High in vitamins B6, C and manganese

Kcal	Carbs	Sugar	Protein	Fat	Sat Fat	Fibre
267	46.9g	32.2g (35.8%)	8.3g	4.1g	1.3g (6.4%)	6.1g (20.4%)

Zesty Quinoa Porridge

Serves 2

Prep. 8 minutes

Vegan

Warm up for your morning training sessions with this citrus-flavoured porridge. Packed full of carbohydrate and B vitamins, which are important for energy metabolism, this is the perfect breakfast to fuel your training. Quinoa has a low glycaemic index (see page 221) releasing energy steadily throughout the day, and it is the only grain that has the full complement of essential amino acids, making it a good protein source. The lemon zest provides a refreshing tang leaving you craving more.

250ml milk, or vegan alternative

80g quinoa, rinsed

1 tsp ground cinnamon

grated zest of 1 lemon

1 tsp sesame seeds

1 tsp chia seeds

1 tsp pumpkin seeds

1. Put the milk in a small saucepan over a medium heat and bring to a simmer. Add the quinoa and return to the boil. Reduce the heat and cook for 15 minutes or until tender.

2. Add the cinnamon and lemon zest to the porridge and stir to combine. Spoon into bowls and top with the seeds. Serve.

Nutrition: Health score 7 High in vitamin B12, copper and manganese

Kcal	Carbs	Sugar	Protein	Fat	Sat Fat	Fibre
480.5	61.4g	17.5g (19.5%)	22.4g	13.2g	3.9g (19.4%)	10g (33.4%)

Ful and Poached Egg

Serves 1

Prep. 15 minutes

Vegetarian, gluten-free

Made with broad beans, herbs and spices, ful is an Egyptian-based dish popular throughout the Middle East as a breakfast option. It is a perfectly balanced meal embracing an impressive array of health benefits including fibre, healthy fats, vitamin B2 and minerals. Give it a go – you won't regret it!

½ tbsp olive oil

200g broad beans, podded fresh or defrosted if frozen

1 garlic clove, crushed, or 1 tsp garlic paste

juice of ½ lemon

½ tbsp tahini paste

1 tsp ground cumin

1 tomato, diced

1 egg

1 tbsp finely chopped parsley

1. Add the olive oil to a pan over a medium heat, then stir in the broad beans, garlic, lemon juice, tahini paste, cumin, tomato and seasoning.

2. Mix well and cook for 9–10 minutes, stirring regularly and gently mashing the mix with a wooden spoon. Stir the chopped parsley through the bean mix once it is cooked.

3. In the meantime, poach the egg. Bring a pan of water at least 5cm deep to boil. Crack the egg into a bowl or saucer and then slide the egg into the water. Cover the pan, turn off the heat and let the egg poach for 4 minutes.

4. To shape the ful mixture, press it into a cylindrical pastry cutter or similar. Serve the egg on top.

Nutrition: Health score 7.8 High in iron, folate and vitamin B2

Kcal	Carbs	Sugar	Protein	Fat	Sat Fat	Fibre
300	18.8g	3.2g (3.6%)	18.2g	14.2g	3g (15%)	8.9g (29.5%)

Carrot Cake Overnight Oats

Serves 1

Prep. 2 minutes

Vegan, gluten-free

Here is the perfect choice for those with a sweet tooth for breakfast cereals, although this version is full of healthy ingredients without being loaded with sugar. This dessert-inspired, all-in-one breakfast provides a whole host of B vitamins for energy, plus vitamin A for good eyesight and blood clotting, and iron for transporting oxygen to power all our cells.

½ carrot, grated

50g (½ cup) porridge oats

3 heaped tbsp chia seeds

a small handful of pecan nuts or walnuts, chopped

a small handful of pumpkin seeds

2 tsp ground cinnamon

1 tsp freshly grated nutmeg

200ml milk, plus extra as needed, or vegan alternative

1 tsp honey (optional)

1. Put the carrot and all the dry ingredients a sealable glass jar and pour in the milk. Seal, and shake until mixed through.
2. Leave to stand for at least 30 minutes or overnight.
3. Add extra milk if needed and honey to taste, if you like, then serve.

Nutrition: Health score 20 High in vitamins A, K and iron

Kcal	Carbs	Sugar	Protein	Fat	Sat Fat	Fibre
653.1	52.2g	23.1g (25.6%)	23.9g	32.1g	7.7g (38.7%)	22.7g (75.8%)

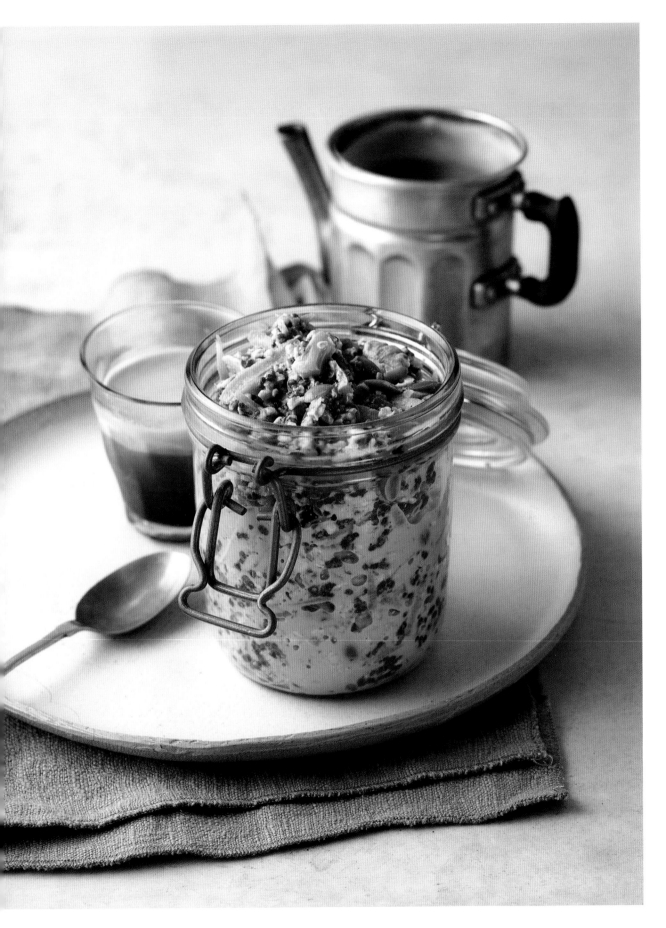

Vanilla and Blueberry Overnight Oats

Serves 1

Prep. 2 minutes

Vegan, gluten-free

My first choice for breakfast is this simple grab-and-go mix for those busy mornings. It provides a combination of protein and carbohydrate to power you through the day, while the blueberries are rich in the phytochemical anthocyanins, a powerful antioxidant, and have anti-inflammatory properties. The chia seeds add healthy fat and a great texture.

50g (½ cup) porridge oats

3 tbsp chia seeds

40g (2 scoops) vanilla protein powder, or vegan alternative

300ml milk, or vegan alternative

3 tbsp natural or Greek yogurt, or vegan alternative

a small handful of blueberries

1 tsp honey (optional), or to taste

1. Put the oats in a sealable glass jar and add the chia seeds, protein powder, milk and 1 tbsp of the yogurt. Seal, and shake until mixed through.

2. Leave to stand for at least 30 minutes or overnight.

2. Spoon over the remaining yogurt and put the blueberries on top. Add the honey and serve.

Nutrition: Health score 15.1 High in vitamin K, manganese and phosphorus

Kcal	Carbs	Sugar	Protein	Fat	Sat Fat	Fibre
581.7	44g	17.7g (19.6%)	40.7g	19.8g	4.6g (22.8%)	19.5g (65%)

Breakfast Burrito

Serves 1

Prep. 5 minutes

Vegetarian

3 eggs, beaten

a handful of spinach

1 wholemeal tortilla wrap

6 baby tomatoes, diced

20g feta cheese, crumbled

Many breakfast options are not balanced meals, but my Mexican-inspired burrito is a rapid breakfast that provides carbs from the tortilla plus protein from the eggs and a range of health benefits.

1. Heat a small saucepan over a medium heat. Pour in the eggs and add the spinach, then cook gently, stirring with a wooden spoon to scramble the eggs. Don't overheat the eggs or they will separate. When just set, remove from the heat, and cover with a lid.

2. Fill the tortilla with the egg, tomatoes and cheese. Roll up, cut in half and serve.

Nutrition: Health score 5.8 High in vitamins B12, A and protein

Kcal	Carbs	Sugar	Protein	Fat	Sat Fat	Fibre
501	38.9g	7.8g (9%)	27g	19g	6.2g (31%)	4.3g (11%)

Almond and Banana Pancakes

Serves 2

Prep. 5 minutes

Vegetarian, gluten-free

1 banana

45g ground almonds

45g (scant ½ cup) porridge oats

75ml almond milk

1 egg

These pancakes taste amazing and have the added health benefits of using banana and oats for the base, as opposed to flour. They provide a good amount of carbs but also some protein, with vitamins B and E thrown in.

1. Put all the ingredients into a food processor or blender and blitz until smooth.

2. Heat a frying pan over a medium heat and add the mixture. Cook for 1 minute or until one side is cooked.

3. Flip over and cook the other side. Serve.

Nutrition: Health score 2.8 High in vitamins B2, E and manganese

Kcal	Carbs	Sugar	Protein	Fat	Sat Fat	Fibre
319	29.9g	10.6g (12%)	11.8g	16.1g	2.3g (12%)	6.3g (17%)

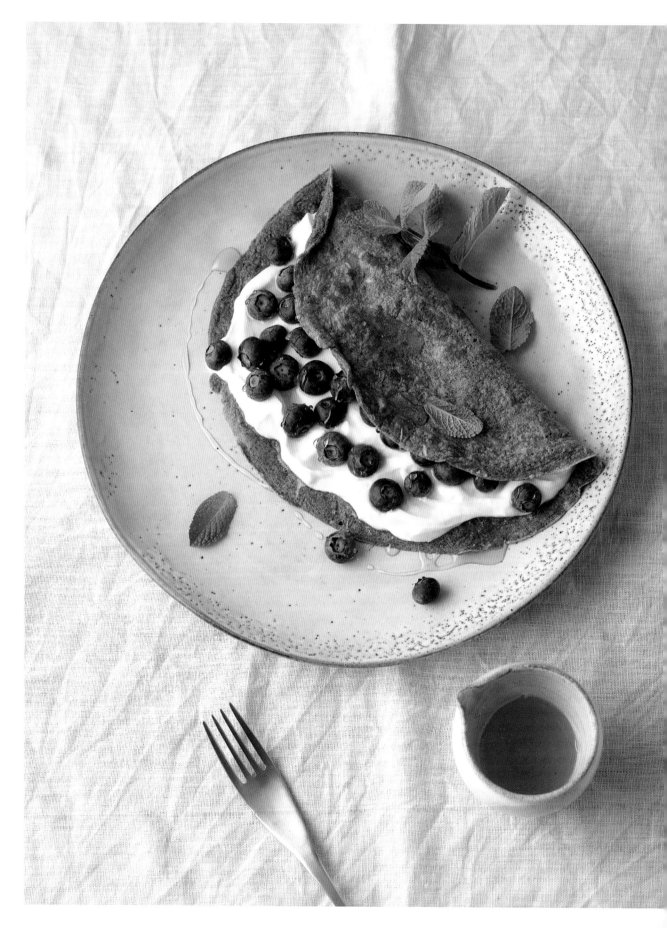

Lean Crêpe

Serves 1

Prep. 8 minutes

Vegetarian, gluten-free

Perfect for those looking to reduce fat mass, these high-protein crêpes are a lower calorie alternative to traditional pancakes, but they still taste amazing with their Greek yogurt and blueberry filling. The blueberries contain anthocyanins, a powerful antioxidant that helps to reduce cell damage, and the yogurt contains probiotics to maintain a healthy gut.

3 eggs, separated, whites only (save the yolks for another recipe)

1 tbsp ground cinnamon

20g (1 scoop) vanilla protein powder

2 tbsp milk

1 tsp olive oil

2 tbsp Greek yogurt

a handful of blueberries

1 tsp honey

1. Put the egg whites in a large grease-free bowl and add the cinnamon, protein powder and milk. Blend or mix well with a whisk or fork.

2. Heat the oil in a frying pan over a medium heat, then pour in mixture. Allow it to spread out, then cook for 2 minutes.

3. Spread the yogurt, berries and honey over half the crêpe, then fold over and serve.

Nutrition: Health score 4.4 High in vitamins B2, B5, D and calcium

Kcal	Carbs	Sugar	Protein	Fat	Sat Fat	Fibre
480	21g	18.5g (21%)	39g	25.3g	12.7g (63%)	3.6g (10%)

Chocolate Orange Pancakes

Serves 2

Prep. 10 minutes

Vegetarian, gluten-free

The traditional combination of chocolate and orange makes these pancakes very popular, but they might seem an unlikely candidate for a healthy breakfast. Nevertheless, they are high in a range of vitamins, minerals, fibre and good fats. Cocoa is not only a lovely rich flavour loved by so many, but it is also healthy, being anti-inflammatory and containing minerals and good fats. The pancakes are fuel based but a still a balanced breakfast with some Lean Muscle and Health. The whole family will gobble them up and they go beautifully with a dollop of Greek yogurt.

80g (¾ cup) porridge oats

125ml milk

1 egg

grated zest of ½ orange

2 tbsp cocoa powder

olive oil (optional)

1. Put all the ingredients, except the oil, into a food processor or blender and blitz until smooth.

2. Either use a non-stick pan or heat a little olive oil in a frying pan over a medium heat. Pour in the mixture to make small pancake shapes in the pan. Cook for 1–2 minutes until golden brown, then carefully flip and cook for a further 1–2 minutes. Transfer to a plate and keep warm. Repeat with the remaining mixture. Serve.

Nutrition: Health score 2 High in iron, manganese and phosphorus

Kcal	Carbs	Sugar	Protein	Fat	Sat Fat	Fibre
199.1	29.2g	11.9 (13.2%)	5.2g	6g	1.1g (5.6%)	4.4g (14.7%)

Banana Breakfast Cookies

Serves 8

Prep. 4 minutes

Vegan

Cookies for breakfast? It's no surprise my kids absolutely gobble these up, but they are healthier than your average cookie because they contain fibre and several minerals. They are an especially good choice for breakfast or a snack when you're on the go and you need to fuel for an active day or sport, as they have a good amount of carbs and potassium from the banana to help with muscle activation.

1 banana

50g (½ cup) porridge oats

70g (½ cup) plain wholemeal flour

½ tsp bicarbonate of soda

2 tbsp peanut butter

1 tbsp agave syrup

2 tbsp dried cranberries

1 tbsp chia seeds

1. Preheat the oven to 200°C (180°C fan oven) Gas 6 and line a baking sheet with baking paper. Put the banana in a bowl and mash using a wooden spoon.

2. Stir in the oats, flour, bicarbonate of soda, peanut butter and syrup.

3. Stir in the cranberries, chia seeds and 25ml water.

4. Put eight spoonfuls of the cookie mixture onto the prepared baking sheet, spacing well apart. Flatten the cookies, then bake for 10 minutes or until golden. Allow to cool or serve warm.

Nutrition: Health score 2 High in iron, manganese and phosphorus

Kcal	Carbs	Sugar	Protein	Fat	Sat Fat	Fibre
199.1	29.2g	11.9g (13.2%)	5.2g	6g	1.1g (5.6%)	4.4g (14.7%)

Smoked Salmon and Guacamole Toast

Serves 1

Prep. 5 minutes

Toast can't be that healthy, can it? Think again! This toast contains over 25 per cent of the recommended dietary amount (RDA) for all your vitamins and minerals, bar three, plus it is high in omega-3 and monounsaturated fats and fibre. It's a brilliantly balanced breakfast containing good amounts of Fuel and Lean Muscle, and bags of Health.

4 cherry tomatoes, cut into quarters

½ small avocado, diced

a squeeze of lime juice

small bunch of fresh coriander, leaves chopped

a pinch of salt

a pinch of ground black pepper

a pinch of dried chilli flakes

2 slices wholemeal bread

2 slices smoked salmon

1. Put the tomatoes and avocado in a bowl

2. Add a squeeze of lime juice, the coriander, salt, pepper and chilli flakes. Mash well, using a fork, to your preferred consistency.

3. Toast the bread, then divide the guacamole between the two slices and top with the smoked salmon. Serve.

Nutrition: Health score 7.4 High in vitamins B6, B12 and selenium

Kcal	Carbs	Sugar	Protein	Fat	Sat Fat	Fibre
412.7	30.7g	5.5g (6.1%)	26.1g	17g	2.8g (14%)	11.1g (37.1%)

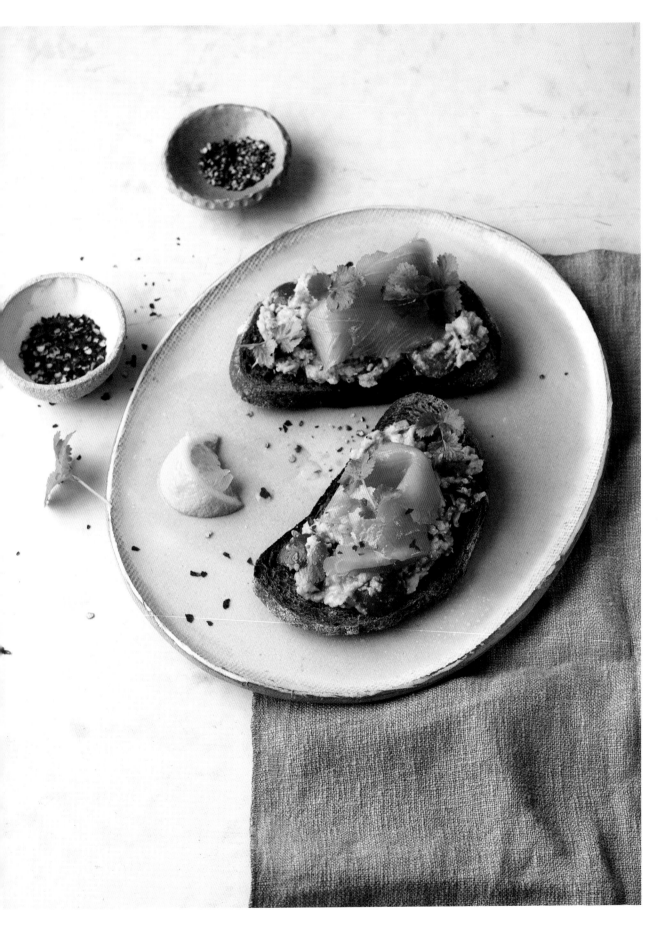

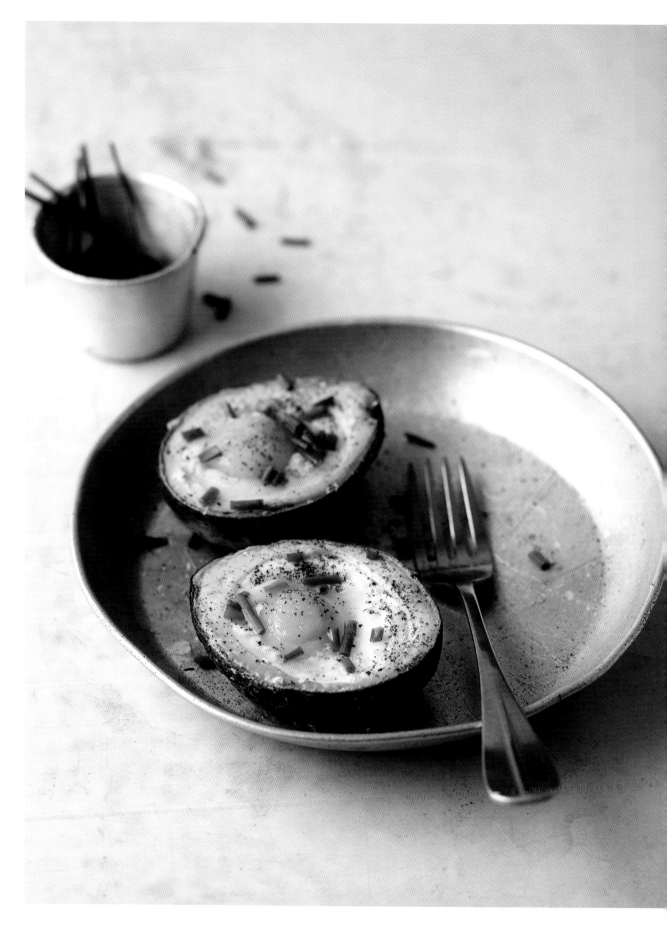

Avocado Baked Eggs

Serves 1

Prep. 4 minutes

Gluten-free, vegetarian

This richly flavoured breakfast is low in carbs and high in protein. The calories are moderate due to the fat content of the eggs and avocado, which is principally monounsaturated and therefore good for health. The avocado and eggs also boast numerous other health benefits for immune function, energy, the skin and bones.

1 avocado

2 eggs

salt and ground black pepper

1 tsp finely chopped chives or spring onions (optional)

1. Preheat the oven to 200°C (180°C fan oven) Gas 6.

2. Cut the avocado in half. Remove the stone and, using a spoon, scoop out a little more in the hollow where the stone was, to accommodate the egg.

3. Put the avocado into an ovenproof dish or ramekin. Crack an egg into each avocado hollow and cook in oven for 10 minutes.

4. Add spring onion or chives, if you like, then serve.

Nutrition: Health score 4.3 High in vitamins B2, K and magnesium

Kcal	Carbs	Sugar	Protein	Fat	Sat Fat	Fibre
382	3.7g	1.5g (1.7%)	15.3g	31.6g	6.2g (31%)	9.3g (24%)

Healthy Mexican Eggs

Serves 2

Prep. 5 minutes

Vegetarian, gluten-free

Caramba! Spice up your morning with this lively breakfast, inspired by Mexican cuisine. The beans are a high-fibre fuel source containing B vitamins, and the eggs add protein and healthy fats, with vitamin C provided by the tomatoes.

1 tbsp olive oil

½ red onion, chopped

2 tomatoes, chopped

1 red chilli, seeded and chopped

3 eggs, lightly beaten

2 tbsp sweet chilli sauce

1 tbsp fresh chopped coriander

1. Heat the oil in a frying pan over a medium heat and fry the diced onion, tomatoes and chilli for 2 minutes.

2. Pour the eggs into the pan and stir constantly with a wooden spoon to scramble them and avoid them sticking. Don't overheat or they will separate. Stir in the chilli sauce and coriander, warm through briefly and serve.

Nutrition: Health score 4.1 High in vitamins A and C

Kcal	Carbs	Sugar	Protein	Fat	Sat Fat	Fibre
230.2	13.2g	10.8g (12%)	10.7g	14.3g	6.3g (15.8%)	3g (10%)

Poached Eggs in Tomato

Serves 2

Prep. 8 minutes

Gluten-free

High in protein and low in carbs, this baked egg dish is great for weight loss or maintenance. It is one of my favourite breakfast options, but you could easily have it as a main meal. Tinned tomatoes are an excellent source of lycopene, shown to help the eyesight and lower the risk of heart disease and prostate cancer.

400g can chopped tomatoes

3 spring onions, finely chopped

handful (30g) of spinach

1 slice (25g) cold meat, sliced

3–4 eggs, according to taste or level of hunger

1. Put the tomatoes in a frying pan over a medium heat and add the spring onions, spinach and meat. Bring to the boil and cook for 2 minutes.

2. Create indentations in the tomatoes with a spoon and crack an egg into each. Bring the mixture to a simmer, then cover the pan with a lid and cook for a further 4 minutes or until the eggs are set. Serve.

Nutrition: Health score 5.7 High in vitamins A, K and selenium

Kcal	Carbs	Sugar	Protein	Fat	Sat Fat	Fibre
220	12.5g	8.1g (9%)	17.3g	10.8g	2.9g (14.9%)	2.7g (9%)

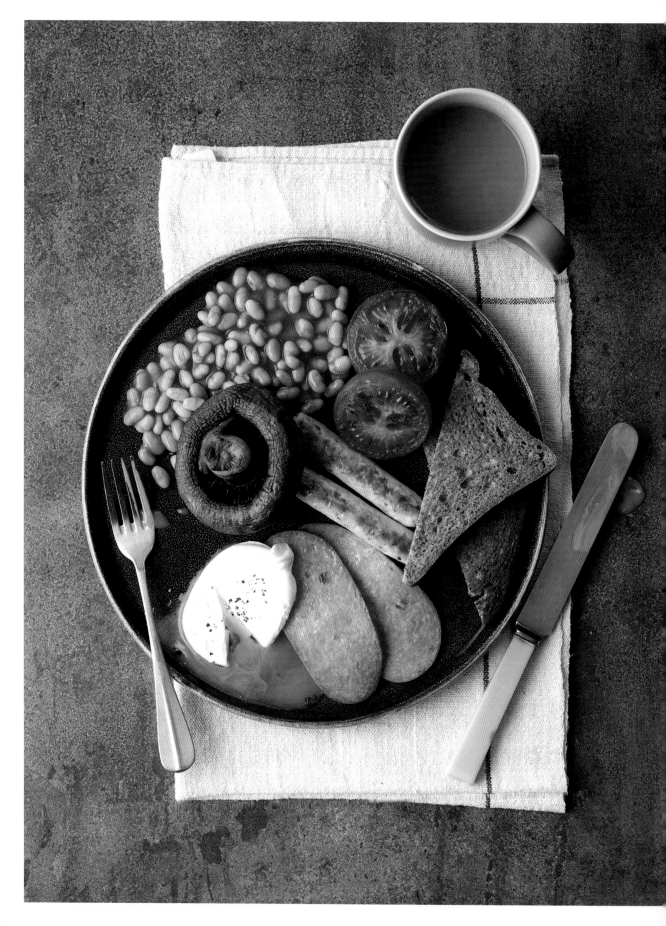

Healthy English Breakfast

Serves 2

Prep. 15 minutes

Vegetarian

This guilt-free English breakfast is the perfect start to any day. It provides a balance of all three macronutrients, and is a healthier alternative to the typical weekend fry-up, as it uses some alternative ingredients and is mostly cooked in the oven. The tomatoes and mushrooms contain the powerful phytochemical, lycopene, which has multiple benefits for a variety of organs in the body, plus the mushrooms also contain prebiotics, which help to keep your gut healthy. What other excuse do you need?

1 tbsp white wine vinegar

4 chicken sausages, or vegan alternative

200g can baked beans

4 turkey-bacon rashers, or vegan alternative

2 portabello mushrooms

2 tomatoes

2 eggs

2 slices brown bread

1. Preheat the oven to 200°C (180°C fan oven) Gas 6, and put a shallow saucepan of boiling water with white wine vinegar on the hob. Bring to the boil and reduce the heat to a simmer.

2. Put the sausages in a roasting pan/grill pan.

3. Meanwhile, put the beans in a saucepan over a medium heat.

4. Cook the sausages according to instructions on the packet.

5. Lightly coat the mushrooms with the olive oil using your fingers or a brush to spread the oil. Halfway through the sausages cooking time add the bacon, mushrooms and tomatoes to the roasting/grill pan, and cook until done.

6. When everything is almost ready, crack the eggs into the simmering water. Poach for 3–4 minutes until done to your liking, then lift out using a slotted spoon.

7. Meanwhile, toast the bread. Serve the eggs with the sausages, bacon, mushrooms and tomatoes, and the toast.

Nutrition: Health score 5.4 High in vitamins B2, B3, D and zinc

Kcal	Carbs	Sugar	Protein	Fat	Sat Fat	Fibre
441	33g	15.4g (17%)	29.7g	18.1g	4.9g (25%)	7.7g (20%)

Courgette Pancakes

Serves 2

Prep. 8 minutes

Vegetarian, gluten-free

For a vegetable slant on a cooked breakfast, try these savoury pancakes. Courgettes are low in calories and high in fibre so, with the addition of the pancake mix being high in protein, they are great for staying lean. The egg and courgette provide a good amount of vitamins A and K, important for blood health.

1 courgette, grated

1 spring onion, finely chopped

1 large egg

2 tbsp coconut oil

salt and ground black pepper

1. Put the courgette in a small bowl and stir in the spring onion.

2. Add the egg to the bowl and mix thoroughly. Season with salt and pepper to taste.

3. Heat the oil in frying pan and spoon three mounds of the courgette mixture into the pan. Fry until lightly browned, pressing down to flatten.

4. Flip the pancakes and cook on the other side until golden. Serve.

Nutrition: Health score 1.7 High in vitamins B12, A and selenium

Kcal	Carbs	Sugar	Protein	Fat	Sat Fat	Fibre
181.9	0.5g	0.5g (0.6%)	4.6g	16.5g	12.2g (60.8%)	0.8g (2.7%)

Breakfast Baustis

Serves 2

Prep. 8 minutes

Gluten-free

Try this tasty variation on the egg theme to make a delicious breakfast. The added chicken makes the dish especially high in protein. The courgette and cauliflower add health benefits and a crunchy texture. You can bake them ahead and eat them for breakfast or a snack on the move.

60g cauliflower, or leftover steamed cauliflower

40g courgette, finely chopped

60g cooked chicken, finely chopped

3 eggs

½ red chilli or chilli flakes (optional)

1. Preheat the oven to 200°C (180°C fan oven) Gas 6 and grease six muffin cups. Lightly steam the cauliflower or use leftover cauliflower. Chop finely.

2. Put the vegetables, chilli (if using) and chicken in a bowl and add 2 eggs. Mix well.

3. Half-fill the muffin cases with the mixture, then bake for 7 minutes.

4. Beat the remaining egg, then add to the top of the muffins. Bake for 7 minutes more, then serve.

Nutrition: Health score 2.4 High in vitamins B12, A and protein

Kcal	Carbs	Sugar	Protein	Fat	Sat Fat	Fibre
170	2.2g	1.8g (2%)	18.7g	8.7g	2.6g (13%)	1.3g (3.5%)

Sweet Potato Hash

Serves 1

Prep. 10 minutes

Vegetarian, gluten-free

Start the day in top form with this warm savoury breakfast. Sweet potato releases energy more steadily than normal potato, sustaining you throughout the morning, and grating it means the dish is cooked in no time. The eggs provide a good source of protein and the onion provides texture and flavour and is anti-inflammatory.

½ onion, chopped

300g sweet potato, coarsely grated

1 tsp olive oil

10g butter

2 eggs

salt and ground black pepper

1. Preheat the oven to 200°C (180°C fan oven) Gas 6. Put the onion in a bowl and mix in the sweet potatoes.

2. Heat the oil and butter in a frying pan over a medium heat, and fry the onion and sweet potato for 4 minutes, turning regularly. Season with salt and pepper.

3. Put the mixture into an ovenproof dish and make two indentations in the mixture. Crack the eggs into the indentations. Cook in the oven for 12 minutes or until eggs are cooked and the hash crispy. Serve.

Nutrition: Health score 8.7 High in vitamins B2, B5 and A

Kcal	Carbs	Sugar	Protein	Fat	Sat Fat	Fibre
488.1	56.7g	15.9g (17.6%)	16.5g	17.7g	8g (40%)	9.8g (32.7%)

Green Shakshuka

Serves 2

Prep. 14 minutes

Vegetarian, gluten-free

Shakshuka is a Middle Eastern and Mediterranean dish where eggs are traditionally poached in a tomato mixture. This version uses green vegetables instead, and the result is not only delicious but also incredibly nutritious, containing over 25 per cent of virtually all your vitamins and minerals, as well as being high in fibre. The eggs and edamame beans provide protein and the various veggies provide low glycaemic carbs (see page 221), making it a winning breakfast or main meal.

1 tbsp olive oil

1 garlic clove, crushed, or 1 tsp garlic paste

1 leek, chopped

80g asparagus, tough ends removed, tips halved

1 tsp ground cumin

1 tbsp ground turmeric

juice of ½ lemon

80g frozen edamame beans

120g baby spinach or chopped kale

2 eggs

1. Heat the oil in a frying pan over a medium heat, then add garlic, leek and asparagus. Cook for 3 minutes, stirring occasionally.

2. Stir in the spices and lemon. Stir in the remaining vegetables and cook for 5 minutes.

3. Use a spoon to create two indentations in the mix. Crack the eggs into the wells and cover with a lid or plate, and cook for a further 5 minutes or until the whites are set and the yolks creamy. Serve

Nutrition: Health score 11.3 High in folate, vitamins A and K

Kcal	Carbs	Sugar	Protein	Fat	Sat Fat	Fibre
248.1	12g	4.2g (4.7%)	14.5g	14.8g	2.8g (14.1%)	6.3g (21%)

Overnight Oats Meal Builder

Overnight oats are my go-to breakfast. They are simple, easy to shape to your goals and easy to transport. Best of all, they are delicious and mega-filling. Preparing your oats in jars is popular because they are so simple to mix and transport, but a bowl works fine.

- Start with the base, which is typically oats or a mix of oats and some nuts or seeds – 70g (½ cup) oats and 4 tablespoons chia seeds is common. Both provide a great texture, fibre and slow-release carbs to sustain us through the morning. Oats have more carbs, and nuts and seeds have more good fats. Bigger is better when it comes to oats, so look for old-fashioned porridge oats. You can also use rolled oats if you prefer a milder taste.

- To add Lean Muscle, protein powder is a convenient choice and can be used to enhance flavour. High-protein yogurts, such as Greek yogurt, are an excellent source of protein and will add a creamy texture.

- Fruit provides great taste and texture, some Fuel and a range of health benefits ranging from vitamins and phytonutrients to fibre. To add some sweetness, cinnamon and cacao are great. Both are high in antioxidants and are anti-inflammatory.

- Finally, we need the milk. Normally, just covering the mixture with milk is about the right quantity and it will typically absorb in about 15 minutes, or you can simply prepare the oats the night before and leave them overnight. Go for dairy or soya milk if you want a bit more protein, or nut milks if you want fewer calories.

PERFORMANCE
FUEL

LEAN
MUSCLE

HEALTH

1. Choose your oats and add to bowl/jar ●

Porridge oats

Rolled

2. Add protein ●

Protein powder

Greek yogurt

Quark

3. Supercharge with healthy fats ●

Chia seeds

Seeds

Nuts

Nut butter

4. Flavour boosters ●

Cinnamon or vanilla

Cacao powder

Honey

Desiccated coconut

5. Add fruit ● ●

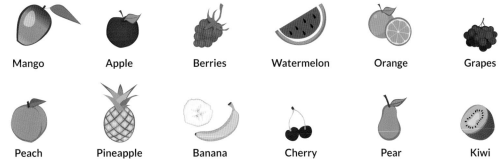

Mango

Apple

Berries

Watermelon

Orange

Grapes

Peach

Pineapple

Banana

Cherry

Pear

Kiwi

6. Cover ingredients with milk ●

7. Mix all ingredients or shake jar, and refrigerate overnight

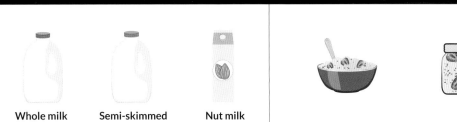

Whole milk

Semi-skimmed

Nut milk

Toast Toppers Meal Builder

I love the smell of toast in the morning; however, plain toast can become a bit mundane and lack protein and healthy nutrients. But, with a bit of imagination, you can transform simple toast into a delicious well-balanced meal that will set you up for the day. I always recommend wholemeal toast, as it is higher in fibre and B vitamins than white.

- After the toast is made, the starting point is to add moisture to the toast and make it sticky to bind other ingredients. Most commonly this would be using butter or margarine, but nut butters have a healthier fat profile and slightly more protein. Pesto and hummus are alternatives and contain good fats. Mashing avocado is a very popular these days – it adds numerous health benefits, some protein and a creamy texture. Mashing banana is also popular, especially for kids, and it adds Fuel and some Health. Cream cheese and cottage cheese are also common and will add some protein.

- To make the toast a more balanced meal, we can now add further toppings. If the topping is moist, such as scrambled egg or tinned tomatoes, you may leave out the initial spread. Eggs are a common choice, be they scrambled, poached or boiled. They are high in protein and numerous nutrients. Smoked salmon and tinned fish, such as mackerel, are high in protein and contain omega-3 fats, which are great for heart and brain health. Other deli meats, such as Parma ham, are a convenient protein source, and vegan options, such a quorn sausages, are a great choice. Baked beans are a toast classic and provide carbs, protein and fibre. Vegetables and fruit, such as tomatoes, spinach and mushrooms, are easy to prepare and add a range of health benefits.

- As a finishing touch to the taste and to garnish, you can sprinkle on any range of spices, oils, herbs or seeds, which will add extra health benefits.

PERFORMANCE
FUEL

LEAN
MUSCLE

HEALTH

Sticky base

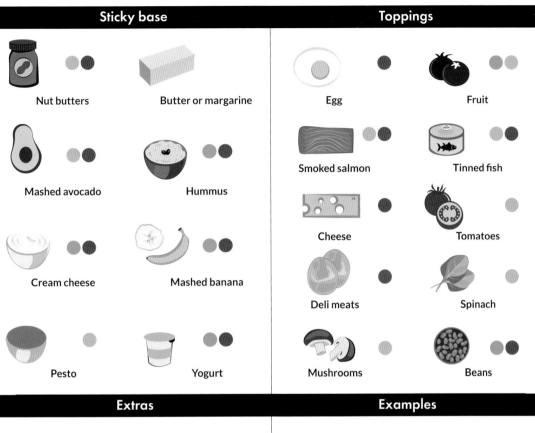

Nut butters

Butter or margarine

Mashed avocado

Hummus

Cream cheese

Mashed banana

Pesto

Yogurt

Toppings

Egg

Fruit

Smoked salmon

Tinned fish

Cheese

Tomatoes

Deli meats

Spinach

Mushrooms

Beans

Extras

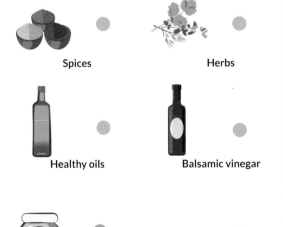

Spices

Herbs

Healthy oils

Balsamic vinegar

Honey

Seeds

Examples

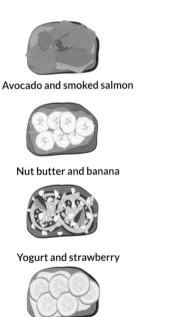

Avocado and smoked salmon

Nut butter and banana

Yogurt and strawberry

Hummus and cucumber

LIGHT MEALS

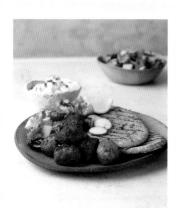

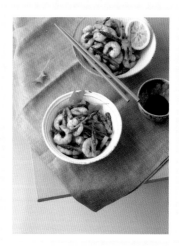

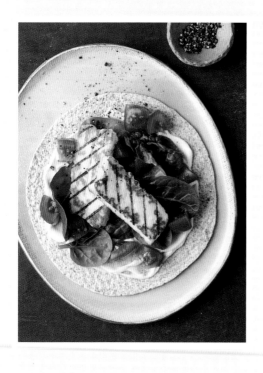

Broccoli and Mint Soup

Serves 2
—
Prep. 8 minutes
—
Vegan, gluten-free
—

Broccoli is known as a super-food for good reason: it has a high level of antioxidants, fibre and potassium. Onions contain the flavonoid allicin, which is anti-inflammatory and lowers blood pressure. The mint adds a fresh flavour to this mega-simple soup.

1 tbsp coconut oil

1 large onion, chopped

1 head of broccoli, cut into florets

700ml chicken or vegetable stock

a small handful of mint leaves

1. Heat the oil in a large saucepan over a medium heat and fry the onion for 5 minutes or until softened.

2. Add the broccoli and stock. Bring to the boil, then reduce the heat and simmer for 10 minutes or until the broccoli has softened.

3. Put in a food processor or blender with the mint leaves and blitz until smooth. Reheat and serve.

Nutrition: Health score 6.1 High in vitamins C and K

Kcal	Carbs	Sugar	Protein	Fat	Sat Fat	Fibre
148.3	13.1g	6.6g (7.3%)	5.4g	7.4g	5.7g (28.6%)	5g (16.8%)

Tuscan Bean Soup

Serves 2

Prep. 10 minutes

Vegan, gluten-free

What better way to warm up in colder weather than with this Tuscan bean soup? It is a perfect for vegetarians and vegans and is packed with half the RDA of fibre, which will keep you feeling full until your next meal as well as being great for gut health. Kale contains high amounts of vitamin C as well. Carrots contain vitamin A, and the onions contain allicin, making this a super-healthy soup.

1 onion, chopped

800ml vegetable stock

a pinch of dried thyme

a pinch of dried oregano

400g can cannellini or haricot beans

400g can chopped tomatoes

3 garlic cloves, crushed, or 3 tsp garlic paste

4 celery sticks, chopped

3 carrots, chopped

2 handfuls of chopped kale

salt and ground black pepper

Put all of the ingredients into a slow cooker. Cook for 8 hours on a low or 3 hours on high. (Alternatively, put all the ingredients in a large saucepan and bring to the boil, reduce the heat and simmer gently for 1 hour.)

Nutrition: Health score 11.7 High in vitamins A, B6, K and iron

Kcal	Carbs	Sugar	Protein	Fat	Sat Fat	Fibre
407.4	56.4g	15.2g (16.8%)	20.6g	3.4g	1.3g (6.5%)	26.9g (56.3%)

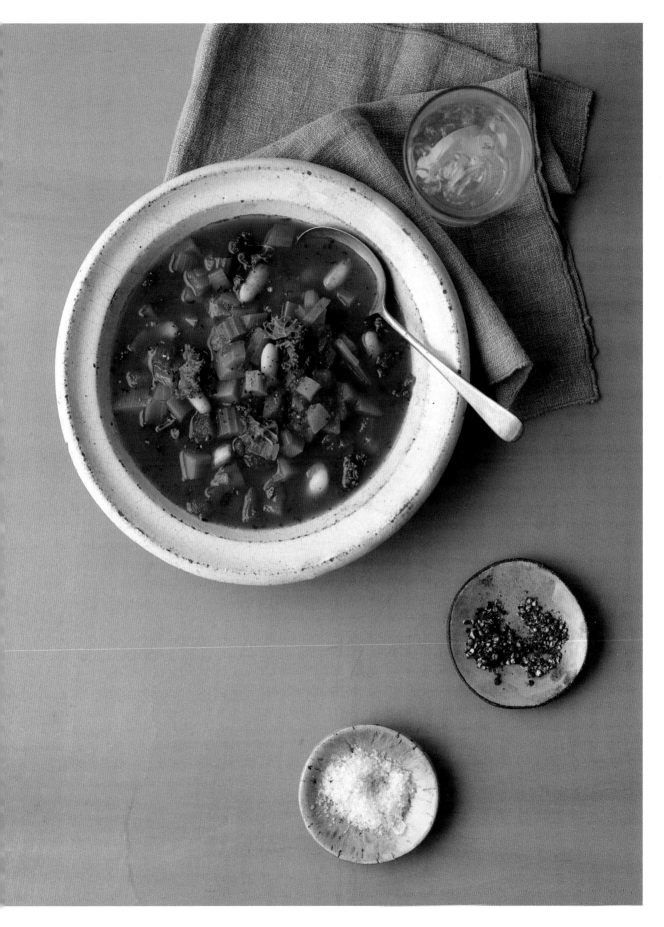

Asian-Style Super Salad

Serves 2

Prep. 10 minutes

Vegan, gluten-free

Full of crunch and fresh Asian flavours, this salad is quick and easy to make and packed with goodness. It is high in important antioxidants vitamin A and C, helping to support the immune system, and vitamin K, which is important for bone health and blood clotting. The ginger adds a moreish zing and has numerous health properties, such being anti-inflammatory.

grated zest and juice of 1 lime

2 tbsp olive oil

1 tsp tamari or soy sauce

20g fresh ginger, peeled and sliced

3 tbsp sesame seeds

½ red cabbage, finely sliced

1 bunch spring onions, finely sliced

2 carrots, grated

3 tsp chia seeds

1. Put the lime zest and juice in a blender or mini-food processor and add the olive oil, soy sauce and ginger. Blitz until smooth.

2. Heat a small saucepan over a low heat and add the sesame seeds. Toast for 1 minute, tossing regularly, until golden. Remove from the heat.

3. Put all the remaining ingredients in a bowl and add the sesame seeds and sauce from the blender. Mix well and serve.

Nutrition: Health score 10 High in vitamins A, B6, C and K

Kcal	Carbs	Sugar	Protein	Fat	Sat Fat	Fibre
239.4	16.2g	8.2g (9.1%)	5.8g	15.5g	2.1g (10.7%)	8.6g (28.6%)

Mango and Pineapple Salad

Serves 4

Prep. 8 minutes

Vegan, gluten-free

Tropical fruits always make a salad particularly refreshing, especially in the summer. Like most salads, this one has numerous health benefits, and clocks up a massive three times the recommended daily allowance (RDA) for vitamin C! It also has a high carb content from the fruit, and so it would support being active. It's definitely one of my favourite salads.

1 ripe mango

1 ripe pineapple, skinned, cored and diced

1 red onion, finely chopped

5 cherry tomatoes

1 red pepper, seeded and diced

2 tbsp chopped fresh coriander

1 red chilli, seeded and finely chopped

juice of 1 lime

2 tbsp olive oil

salt and ground black pepper

1. Using a sharp knife, cut each side of the mango away from the large pit in the centre. Score squares into the mango flesh and then push the skin side inwards to make the mango cubes stand proud. Cut off the cubes. Cut off the flesh around the pit and dice it.

2. Put the mango in a salad bowl and add the pineapple, onion, tomatoes and red pepper. Add the coriander, chilli, lime juice and oil. Season with salt and pepper, then mix well. Serve.

Nutrition: Health score 8.3 High in vitamins B6, C, K and and potassium

Kcal	Carbs	Sugar	Protein	Fat	Sat Fat	Fibre
275.2	46.3g	40.4g (44.9%)	3.9g	7.8g	1.1g (5.5%)	7.4g (19.5%)

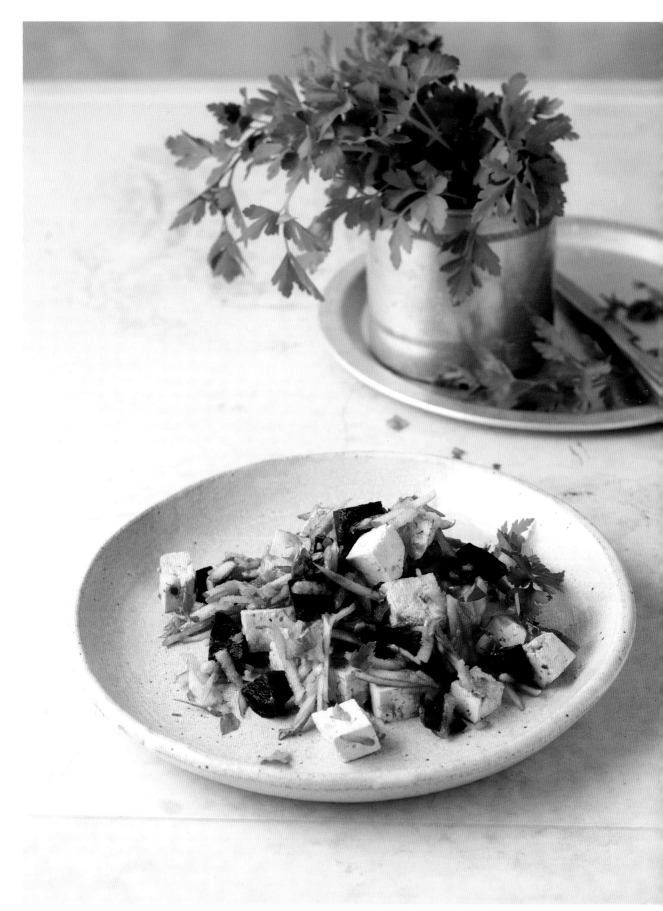

Beetroot and Apple Salad with Smoked Tofu

Serves 1

Prep. 10 minutes

Vegan, gluten-free

The sweet combination of beetroot and apple goes very well with smoked tofu in this vegan salad that is simple but out of the ordinary with its different textures and flavours. The smoked tofu provides protein; the beetroots provide nitrates, which boost energy production via dilating blood vessels, and are anti-ageing; and the apples are high in fibre and antioxidants.

2 cooked beetroots, chopped into cubes

1 dessert apple, cored, peeled and grated

1 garlic clove, crushed, or 1 tsp garlic paste

100g smoked tofu, cut into small cubes

1 tbsp olive oil

salt and ground black pepper

Put all the ingredients in a salad bowl, season with salt and pepper, and mix well. Serve.

Nutrition: Health score 5.7 High in manganese, vitamin K and selenium

Kcal	Carbs	Sugar	Protein	Fat	Sat Fat	Fibre
364.7	33.6g	29.9g (33%)	12.9g	17.7g	2.5g (12.7%)	9.4g (24.8%)

Easy Tuna Salad

Serves 1

Prep. 10 minutes

Gluten-free

Sometimes the easiest things are the best, and this tuna salad is just right for a quick lunch that ticks all the right health boxes. The moderate calorie load and high protein content make it a great choice for staying lean. It has a high health score with a range of nutrients important for energy metabolism, immunity, and healthy skin and bones.

2 eggs

50g mixed salad leaves

2 tomatoes, quartered

½ onion, finely chopped

100g can tuna, drained

10 pitted olives, halved

1 tsp pepper

1 tbsp olive oil

1 tsp chopped fresh basil, or to taste

1. Put the eggs in a saucepan of boiling water. Return to the boil and cook for 10 minutes. Drain the pan and refill with cold water. Drain and fill again. Leave the eggs to cool, then cut into quarters.

2. Put the salad leaves in a serving bowl and add the tomatoes.

3. Put the onion in a bowl and add the tuna and olives. Season with the pepper and mix well. Put the tuna on top of the salad and drizzle over the olive oil. Add the eggs and sprinkle with basil. Serve.

Nutrition: Health score 9.1 High in vitamins A, B3 and B12

Kcal	Carbs	Sugar	Protein	Fat	Sat Fat	Fibre
486	11.3g	8.5g (9.5%)	47.1g	26.3g	5.4g (26.9%)	3.7g (12.4%)

Spanish Tomato Salad

Serves 2

Prep. 10 minutes

Vegan

Let the flavours of Spain embrace you in this easy-to-make vegan salad. Tomatoes are a Spanish classic, and they are full of vitamin C to boost immunity, and vitamin K, which is important for heart health. The bread adds a nice crunch and adds Fuel, making this a good choice when active.

60g ciabatta, cut into slices

1 small onion, sliced

1 garlic clove, crushed, or 1 tsp garlic paste

½ small bunch of parsley, leaves chopped

1 tbsp lemon juice

2 tbsp olive oil

1 tsp salt

1 tsp ground black pepper

500g mixed tomatoes, sliced

½ cucumber, sliced

1. Preheat the oven to 190°C (170°C fan oven) Gas 5. Put the ciabatta on a baking tray and bake for 10 minutes, then allow to cool and cut into large croutons.

2. Put the onion in a small bowl and cover with cold water. Leave to soak for 30 minutes.

3. Put the garlic in a small bowl and add the parsley, lemon juice, olive oil, salt and pepper. Mix well.

4. Put the tomatoes in a serving dish and add the cucumber. Drain the onion and add to the bowl. Add the dressing and toss well. Top with the croutons and serve.

Nutrition: Health score 8.6 High in vitamins A, C and iron

Kcal	Carbs	Sugar	Protein	Fat	Sat Fat	Fibre
445.3	27.1g	11.7g (13%)	6.2g	15.5g	2.1g (10.5%)	5.8g (19.3%)

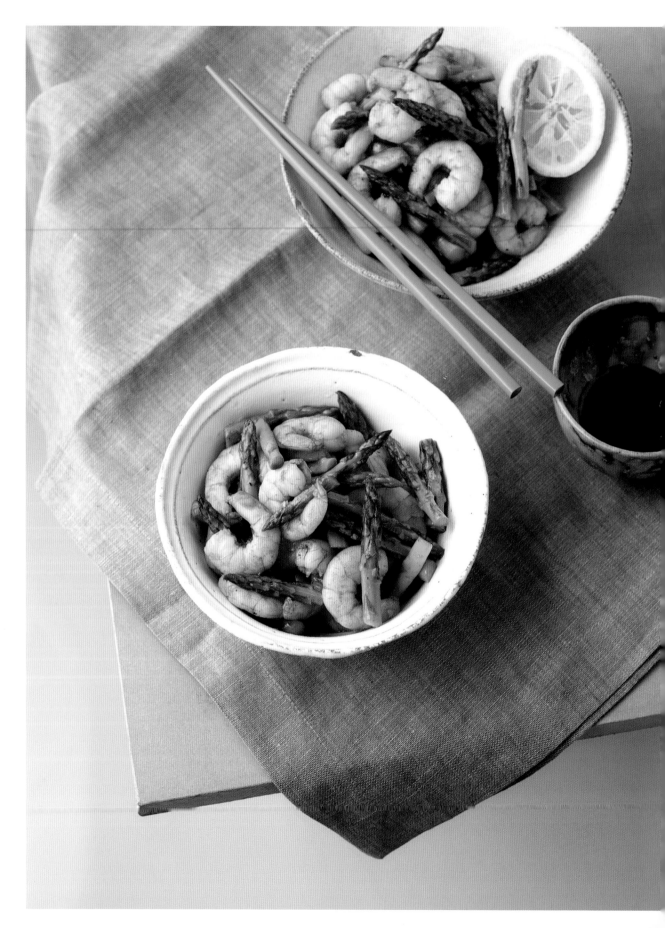

Prawn and Asparagus Stir-Fry

Serves 2

Prep. 12 minutes

Gluten-free

This super-quick stir-fry is very low in carbs and calories, making it the perfect choice for those looking to lose weight. It could easily be combined with noodles if you wanted a bit more of a carb and calorie punch. Prawns are a great source of B vitamins and protein, and asparagus is high in fibre, vitamin C and the antioxidants, glutathione and rutin.

4 tsp olive oil

500g raw shelled prawns

1 tbsp paprika, Cajun seasoning or crushed red pepper flakes

2–3 cloves garlic, to taste, crushed, or 2–3 tsp garlic paste

500g asparagus, tough ends removed, chopped

5cm fresh ginger, peeled and grated

1 tbsp tamari or light soy sauce

juice of 1 lemon

1. Heat 2 teaspoons of the oil in a frying pan over a medium-high heat. Add the prawns, paprika and 1 garlic clove. Cook until the prawns are pink and cooked through. Remove from the pan.

2. Add 2 teaspoons of oil to the pan. Add the asparagus followed by the remaining garlic and the ginger. Cook for 3 minutes, then add the prawns. Add the tamari or soy sauce and lemon juice. Cook for 1 minute and serve.

Nutrition: Health score 8.7 High in vitamins B3, A and copper

Kcal	Carbs	Sugar	Protein	Fat	Sat Fat	Fibre
251.9	4.9g	3.4g (3.8%)	44.6g	5.5g	0.8g (4.2%)	4.4g (11.6%)

Almond-Breaded Chicken Strips

Serves 2

Prep. 5 minutes

Gluten-free

These chicken strips are a great healthy alternative to breadcrumbed and fried chicken, and they taste amazing. They predominantly provide lean protein, but the almonds also contain healthy fats and vitamin E. Oven baking rather than deep-frying keeps the calories and saturated fat to a minimum.

200g ground almonds

1 tsp onion powder

1 tbsp chopped fresh parsley

2 skinless chicken breasts, cut into strips

3 eggs, beaten

olive oil spray

salt and ground black pepper

1. Preheat the oven to 200°C (180°C fan oven) Gas 6. Put the ground almonds in a large bowl and add the onion powder and parsley. Season with salt and pepper and mix well.

2. Dip the chicken strips into the almond mixture, then into the beaten egg. Then dip back into the almond mixture. Put on a baking sheet.

3. Spray with oil and then bake for 25–30 minutes, turning after 15 minutes, until golden. Serve.

Nutrition: Health score 4.6 High in vitamin B3, B6 and selenium

Kcal	Carbs	Sugar	Protein	Fat	Sat Fat	Fibre
411.4	3.4g	1.6g (1.7%)	47.3g	21.5g	3.7g (18.7%)	3.2g (10.6%)

Tortilla Pizza

Serves 1

Prep. 5 minutes

Everyone loves a pizza! The difference here is that this tortilla pizza is packed full of nutrients and provides a balance of protein, carbohydrate and micronutrients in a low-calorie alternative to a takeaway. You can easily customise your pizza by using a variety of toppings to meet your preferences. It's also a great dish to get the kids involved in preparing and cooking to foster an interest in healthy eating.

1 large soft wholemeal tortilla wrap

2 tbsp passata sauce

1 tbsp chopped fresh parsley or coriander

a small handful of grated low-fat cheese

1–2 slices lean meat (such as chicken, turkey, ham)

your choice of toppings (such as sliced red chilli, sliced mushrooms, sliced peppers)

a large handful of baby spinach leaves

1. Preheat the oven to 200°C (180°C fan oven) Gas 6. Put the tortilla wrap on a baking sheet. Spoon the passata evenly over the wrap and sprinkle the herbs on top.

2. Scatter the cheese over the top and add your choice of lean meat and toppings.

3. Put the spinach in a colander and pour over boiling water to wilt it, then rinse it in cold water. Add to the pizza. Bake for 12–15 minutes. Serve.

Nutrition: Health score 5.1 High in vitamins A, B3, B6 and K

Kcal	Carbs	Sugar	Protein	Fat	Sat Fat	Fibre
479.4	50.3g	19.1g (21.2%)	43.5g	8.9g	3.2g (15.9%)	7.8g (25.8%)

Falafels

Serves 2

Prep. 12 minutes

Vegan

Falafels are a delicious Middle-Eastern-derived dish made with chickpeas, herbs and spices. In Western culture, they are often added to pitta bread as an amazing street food that I often hunt out at festivals. The chickpea base means that they are Fuel dominant. They have an impressive Health content, being high in copper, iron and phosphorus, in addition to being high in fibre and monounsaturated fats. Protein is also quite high at over 12g per serving.

400g can chickpeas, drained and rinsed

3 garlic cloves

1 onion, roughly chopped

1 small handful of fresh parsley, leaves only

1 tsp ground coriander

½ tsp ground cumin

½ tsp salt

2 tbsp plain flour

4 tbsp olive oil

1. Put all the ingredients, except the oil, in a food processor or blender and blitz until smooth.

2. Shape the mixture into small balls.

3. Heat the oil in a frying pan over a medium heat and cook the falafel for 2 minutes on one side them, flip them and fry the other side for 2 minutes or until cooked through and golden.

Nutrition: Health score 5.5 High in folate, vitamin K and iron

Kcal	Carbs	Sugar	Protein	Fat	Sat Fat	Fibre
489.4	33.5g	8.2g (9.1%)	12.6g	30.6g	4.1g (20.6%)	11g (36.6%)

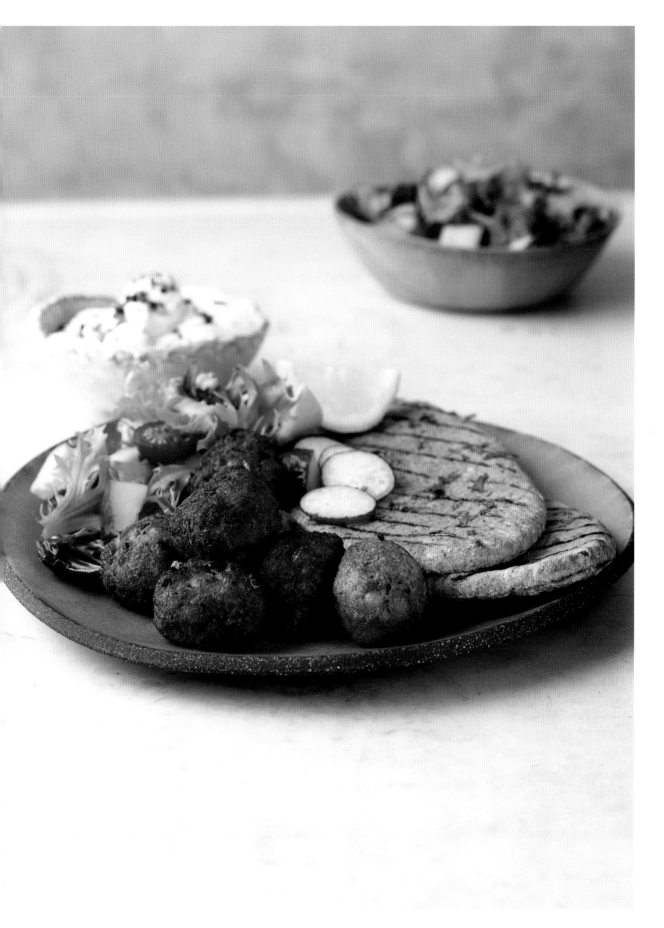

Mediterranean Wrap

Serves 1

Prep. 6 minutes

Tuna combines with avocado and red pepper to make a well-flavoured filling for a wrap. It is protein rich to appease hunger, and it contains heart-healthy monounsaturated fatty acids and an array of B vitamins that promote the efficient metabolism of energy within our muscle cells. The tortilla wrap provides Fuel to make this a perfectly balanced meal for all occasions.

½ avocado

juice of ½ lemon

1 soft wholemeal tortilla wrap

200g can tuna, drained

2 tsp vinaigrette, or light salad dressing

½ onion, finely sliced

8cm cucumber, sliced

½ green pepper, finely chopped

1 tbsp fresh chopped coriander

ground black pepper

1. Scoop the avocado into a small bowl and mash with a fork. Add the lemon juice and mix well, then spread the mix on the wrap.

2. Put the tuna in a bowl and add the vinaigrette, onion, cucumber, green pepper and coriander. Season with black pepper. Mix together well.

3. Fill the tortilla wrap with the tuna mixture. Fold up the bottom of the wrap and then fold over the sides to form a cylinder. Serve.

Nutrition: Health score 10.4 High in vitamins A, K and sodium

Kcal	Carbs	Sugar	Protein	Fat	Sat Fat	Fibre
515	38.1g	9.3g (10.3%)	42.8g	16.7g	2.4g (12.1%)	14.8g (49.4%)

Ham, Egg and Avocado Wrap

Serves 1

Prep. 10 minutes

2 eggs

½ red onion, thinly sliced

½ avocado, sliced

a handful of baby spinach

5 cherry tomatoes

2 soft wholemeal tortilla wraps

2 slices cooked ham

Make this simple but tasty wrap with salad that you have in the fridge. It packs an impressive protein punch through the ham, eggs and avocado, which also contains healthy fats and adds a lovely creamy texture.

1. Put the eggs in a saucepan of boiling water. Return to the boil and cook for 10 minutes. Drain the pan and refill with cold water. Drain and fill again. Leave the eggs to cool, then chop.

2. Layer the salad (onion, avocado, spinach and tomatoes) over the tortilla wrap. Top with the ham and the chopped boiled egg, then fold up. Slice and serve.

Nutrition: Health score 4 High in vitamins A, B2 and K

Kcal	Carbs	Sugar	Protein	Fat	Sat Fat	Fibre
365.4	38.2g	4.9g (5.4%)	16.9g	14.5g	4.1g (20.3%)	6g (19.9%)

Peanut Butter and Banana Wrap

Serves 1

Prep. 2 minutes

Vegan

1 banana

2 tbsp peanut butter

1 soft wholemeal tortilla wrap

Quick and easy to make, the filling for this wrap might take you back to your childhood. The high calories and carb content make it a great fuel choice. The peanut butter adds healthy monounsaturated fats.

1. Mash the banana with a fork.

2. Spread the peanut butter over the centre of the wrap and top with the mashed banana. Roll up and cut in half. Serve.

Nutrition: Health score 3.3 High in vitamins B3, B6 and manganese

Kcal	Carbs	Sugar	Protein	Fat	Sat Fat	Fibre
596.3	65.2g	21.5g (23.9%)	17.7g	29.8g	6.9g (34.7%)	8.3g (27.6%)

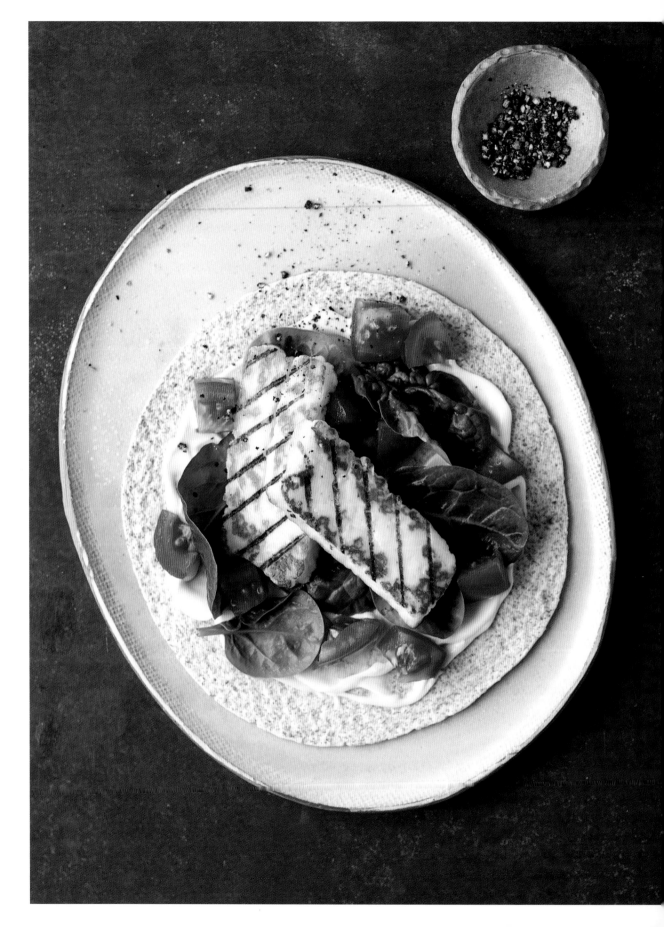

Grilled Halloumi Wrap

Serves 2

Prep. 10 minutes

Vegetarian

This wrap is absolutely delicious because of the salty moreishness of the halloumi. This firm cheese has an incredible flavour and texture, and it is higher in protein than most cheeses. The wrap also makes it a suitable fuel choice, and there are good levels of vitamins A, C and K, and folate, making it a winner all round.

125g low-fat halloumi

1 tomato, chopped

2 soft wholemeal tortilla wraps

2 handfuls of baby spinach

mayonnaise (optional)

black pepper to taste

1. Preheat the grill to high. Slice the halloumi into four even-width rectangular pieces. Grill the halloumi for 4 minutes on each side until slightly charred.

2. Spread each wrap with a little mayo, if using, put half the tomato on each, along with a handful of spinach.

3. Put two halloumi slices on each wrap and sprinkle with pepper. Serve.

Nutrition: Health score 2.5 High in vitamins A, K and sodium

Kcal	Carbs	Sugar	Protein	Fat	Sat Fat	Fibre
524.8	33.8g	6.6g (7.3%)	28g	29.5g	17.6g (88.2%)	5.8g (19.4%)

Salad Meal Builder

Salads are simple, extremely nutritious, easy to transport and, with a bit of imagination, can be mega-tasty. Their uncooked nature means that the ingredients often retain their highest nutritional value. Salads are associated with health but can be a great source of fuel and protein.

- If you are cooking any of your protein sources, then this is usually the starting point. Similarly, if you are adding a grain-type carb that is not quick-cook, you may need to prepare it slightly earlier. It is personal preference as to whether you leave to cool or add to the salad warm.
- There is no defined order, but salad items normally form the base of the dish, especially if you are using green leaves such as spinach, lettuce and rocket. Peel and chop the salad and vegetables as necessary. Although not shown on the infographic, fruits can really make a dish, but they are seldom used in salads (mango is my favourite).
- To add fuel, quick-cook wholemeal rice and pasta, couscous and quinoa are good choices, as is any type of canned beans.
- Add your cooled or warm protein, such as egg, tinned fish or tofu.
- Garnishes add extra flavour and nutrients. Nuts and seeds are a source of good fats and add a pleasing texture.
- The finishing and most important touch, is the dressing. It can be as simple as oil, balsamic vinegar or lemon juice, and you will see some great homemade sauces in the graphic. Beware: some pre-made salad sauces can be very high in sugar.

PERFORMANCE
FUEL

LEAN
MUSCLE

HEALTH

1. Add salad and vegetable items

Leaves, lettuce, rocket   **Spinach**   **Peppers**   **Carrots**   **Broccoli**   **Onion**   **Chilli**

Cucumber   **Tomato**   **Aubergine**   **Beetroot**   **Corn**   **Olives**   **Cabbage**

2. Choose your carbs

Rice brown, basmati   **Quinoa, buckwheat**   **Beans** chickpeas, black, kidney, mung

Wholewheat pasta   **Couscous**

3. Pick a protein

Cold meats chicken, turkey, ham   **Tinned fish** tuna, kipper, sardines   **Prawns**

Cooked meats chicken, turkey, beef etc   **Eggs**   **Tofu**

4. Add healthy fats

Avocado   **Seeds** pumpkin, chia, flax, sunflower, sesame   **Hummus**   **Nuts** walnut, almond, cashew, pine

5. Garnish for flavour

Fresh herbs   **Chives**   **Fruit** mango, berries, apple, peach, etc

6. Add dressing

Pre-made hot sauce, sweet chilli, Thai, mango and chilli, honey and mustard

Balsamic

Virgin oil

Lemon yogurt 1 garlic clove, 2 tbsp lemon juice, 1 tsp mustard, 2 tbsp yogurt, 2 tbsp oil

Lemon and chilli ½ lemon juice, sliced chilli, 2 tbsp olive oil

Wrap and Sandwich Builder

Explaining how to make a sandwich might seem like teaching you to suck eggs, but most of us make the same one or two types of sandwiches all the time. This builder will help you to mix things up and meet your nutritional goals.

- Bread is the obvious staring point and I would always recommend wholemeal for extra fibre and vitamins. The saying 'white bread – you're dead' has always stuck with me, although a little dramatic! Thicker breads, such as subs, will provide the most fuel and calories, and thinner breads like pittas and tortillas, the least.

- The order of filling a sandwich is not that important. For some recipes you would chop and add everything to a bowl and mix before adding as a filling, and this works great with wraps. If you are using a sticky topping like guacamole, however, it's sometimes useful to put that on first so that you can put in on the bread base and it can help to bind the other ingredients.

- Lean Muscle protein choices are many and varied. You can buy cured meats or cook your own. Canned fish is also a great choice.

- Your Health choices come from the array of salad items (and you can add pickled veg) that normally top the filling. Many of us stick to lettuce and cucumber, but think bolder and a greater range of colours, such as baby spinach, beetroot and tomato for maximum health benefits and taste.

- The final sauce or dressing is where things can take a downturn, as many are high in fat, sugar and salt. Opt for lower-fat versions where possible – but be careful that the fat hasn't been replaced by sugar – or make your own. There are some good examples in the infographic.

PERFORMANCE
FUEL

LEAN
MUSCLE

HEALTH

1. Choose your bread

Wholemeal wrap

Wholemeal pitta

Wholemeal sub

Granary/seeded bread

2. Fill with protein

Cold or cooked meats, chicken, turkey, ham, lean beef, salmon, prawns

Tinned fish
tuna, kippers, sardines

Eggs

Tofu or tempeh

Beans
chickpeas, black, kidney, mung

3. Add salad and vegetable items

Lettuce

Spinach

Carrots

Cucumber

Onion

Chilli

Tomato

Peppers

Beetroot

Sweetcorn

Olives

Cabbage

4. Add optional deli item

Avocado

Feta/mozzarella

Hummus

Serrano ham

5. Garnish for flavour

Herbs
mint, basil, parsley, coriander

Chives

6. Sauce it up

Pre-made
hot sauce, sweet chilli, Thai, mango and chilli, honey and mustard, light mayo

Curried yogurt
1 tbsp lemon juice, 2 tbsp yogurt, ½ tsp curry powder

Salsa
2 tomatoes, ¼ small onion, 1 chilli (all diced), 1 tbsp lime juice

Guacamole
1 avocado, ½ tomato, (finely diced), 1 tbsp chilli flakes, 2 tbsp lime juice

MAIN MEALS

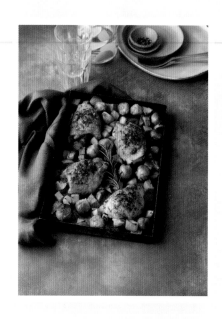

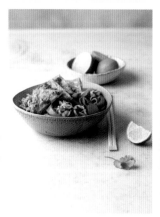

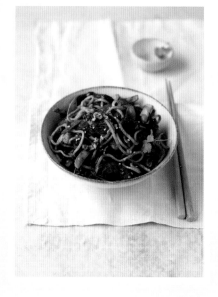

Lemon Pasta with Courgette and Tomato

Serves 1

Prep. 15 minutes

Vegan

Ready in no time, this light and zingy pasta dish is a great choice for vegans, when made with a vegan yogurt and cheese. Although it is Fuel dominant to support activity, it has a balance of all three macronutrients and is low in fat due to its yogurt base. The courgette and tomato add vibrant colours with varied phytonutrients and fibres.

50g wholegrain spaghetti, or other pasta

45g Greek yogurt, or vegan alternative

30g Parmesan, or vegan alternative, grated

grated zest and juice of ½ lemon

2 tsp olive oil

1 courgette, diced

1 garlic clove, finely chopped, or 1 tsp garlic paste

1 large tomato, sliced

salt and ground black pepper

1. Cook the spaghetti in a saucepan of boiling water for 8–10 minutes, or according to the pack instructions, until the pasta is tender but with a bite. Drain in a colander, then return it to the pan.

2. Add the yogurt, Parmesan, lemon zest and juice, and season with salt and pepper. Mix thoroughly.

3. Heat the oil in a large saucepan over a medium heat and cook the courgette until softened, turning occasionally.

4. Make a space in the pan by pushing the courgette to one side then add the garlic and tomato slices. Cook for 15–30 seconds.

5. Transfer the courgette mixture to the pan with the pasta mixture and stir gently until combined. Serve.

Nutrition: Health score 5.3 High in vitamins A, C, calcium and potassium

Kcal	Carbs	Sugar	Protein	Fat	Sat Fat	Fibre
480.6	45.8g	10.3g (11.4%)	20.6g	22.7g	8g (39.9%)	8.3g (21.9%)

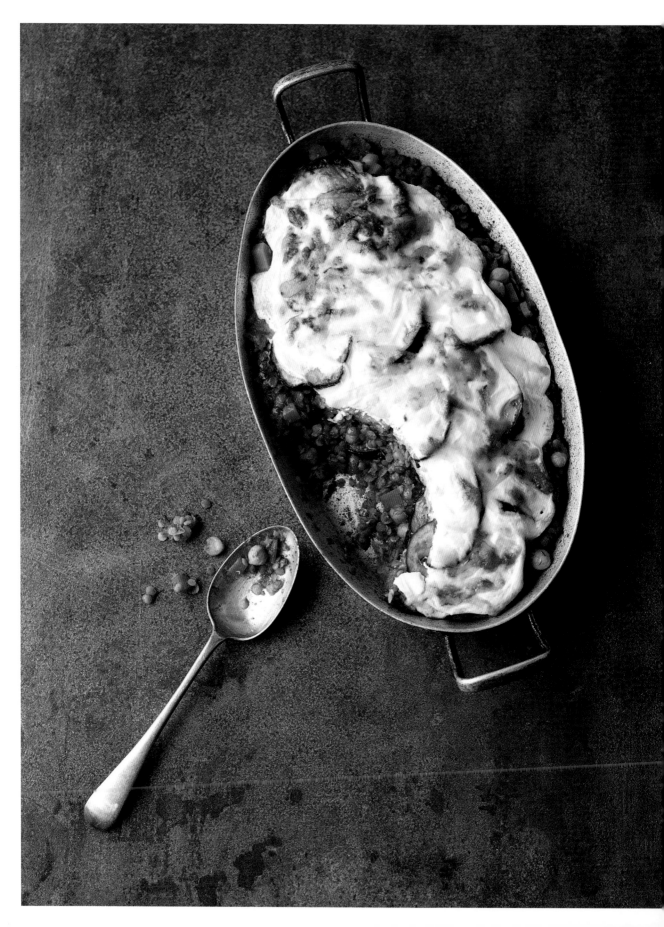

Aubergine and Lentil Bake

Serves 3

Prep. 20 minutes

Vegan, gluten-free

This dish is one of the main reasons I started to embrace vegan cooking. Although you can use dairy products to make it, it also tastes utterly delicious with vegan yogurt and cheese. It is carb-dominant, but it also provides a great dose of protein. It offers a vast array of vitamins and minerals and has one of the highest health scores within the Colour-Fit library.

1 tbsp olive oil, plus extra for shallow frying

1 onion, chopped

1 celery stick, chopped

1 carrot, chopped

1 tsp chilli powder

1 tsp ground cumin

1 tsp ground cinnamon

1 tsp smoked paprika

1 garlic clove, crushed, or 1 tsp garlic paste

400g can chopped tomatoes

3 tbsp tomato purée

400g can chickpeas, drained and rinsed

175g red lentils

1 aubergine, thickly sliced

300g low-fat Greek yogurt or vegan alternative

50g reduced-fat Cheddar cheese or vegan alternative, grated

1. Preheat the oven to 180°C (160°C fan oven) Gas 4. Heat the 1 tbsp oil in a saucepan over a medium-low heat and cook the onion, carrot and celery for 5 minutes, then add the spices and garlic. Cook for a further 2–3 minutes.

2. Add the chopped tomatoes, tomato purée, chickpeas and lentils. Stir and bring to the boil, then reduce the heat to a simmer.

3. Heat a frying pan with a thin film of oil over a medium-high heat, and fry the aubergine slices until slightly golden on both sides.

4. Put a layer of the tomato mixture into an ovenproof dish, then add a layer of aubergine, repeating the process until 1cm from the top of the dish.

5. Spread the yogurt over the top and sprinkle with cheese. Bake for 30 minutes, then serve.

Nutrition: Health score 13.5 High in vitamins B1, A and folate

Kcal	Carbs	Sugar	Protein	Fat	Sat Fat	Fibre
642	78.5g	25.1g (27.8%)	46.1g	7.3g	1.5g (7.6%)	28.7 g (95.6%)

Huevos Rancheros

Serves 2

Prep. 12 minutes

Vegetarian, gluten-free

This traditional Mexican meal is an absolute nutritional powerhouse, because it contains over 25 per cent of virtually all your micronutrients and is high in healthy monounsaturated fat. Although it is often used as a breakfast, the balance of carbs from the beans and protein from the eggs make it a perfect meal any time. Added to that, it is absolutely delicious – you'd be *loco* not to try it!

1 tbsp olive oil

1 red onion, chopped

1 tsp ground cumin

1 tsp dried chilli flakes

juice of ½ lemon

400g can black beans, drained and rinsed

2 eggs

1 avocado

salt and ground black pepper

1. Heat the oil in a saucepan over a medium heat, add the onion and cook for 3 minutes.

2. Add the spices and lemon juice, and stir to mix, then add black beans and cook for 4 minutes. Season with salt and pepper.

3. While the beans are cooking, put a shallow saucepan of boiling water over a medium-high heat. Return to a simmer. Crack the eggs into the simmering water and poach for 3–4 minutes until done to your liking.

4. Cut the avocado in half, remove the pit and scoop out the inside using a spoon. Slice the flesh. Divide the bean mixture between two plates and top with the avocado. Lift out the eggs using a slotted spoon and place on the avocado. Serve.

Nutrition: Health score 9.1 High in vitamin B1, folate and iron

Kcal	Carbs	Sugar	Protein	Fat	Sat Fat	Fibre
583.7	41.5g	9.2g (10.3%)	26.1g	24g	4.1g (20.7%)	30.4g (101.2%)

Chickpea Chaat

Serves 4

Prep. 10 minutes

Vegan, gluten-free

Sweetcorn and chickpeas make this vegan curry high in Fuel with a massive hit of flavours and textures. It packs an impressive 23g of protein per serving – unusual for a vegan dish. The range of veggies, fruit and salad means that it possesses numerous health benefits, due to its range of vitamins, minerals and high fibre content.

2 tbsp olive oil

½ red onion finely chopped

1 red chilli, seeded and chopped

8 cherry tomatoes

1 handful of fresh coriander, leaves chopped

1 handful of fresh mint, leaves chopped

grated zest and juice of 1 lime

1 tsp garam masala

100g cucumber, diced

4 tbsp pomegranate seeds

400g can chickpeas, drained and rinsed

300g can sweetcorn, drained and rinsed

1. Heat 1 tbsp of the oil in a small saucepan and fry the onion and half the chilli for 2 minutes. Add the tomatoes and fry for a further 2 minutes, then leave to cool.

2. Put the remaining chilli into a food processor or blender and add the herbs, lime zest and juice and 1 tbsp olive oil. Blitz until smooth.

3. Put the fried mixture into a bowl and add the herb dressing and the remaining ingredients. Mix together well. Serve.

Nutrition: Health score 8.7 High in folate, vitamin C and iron

Kcal	Carbs	Sugar	Protein	Fat	Sat Fat	Fibre
569.8	70.9g	27.3g (30.3%)	23.4g	14.8g	1.9g (9.7%)	21.7g (72.2%)

Black Bean Burgers

Serves 4

Prep. 20 minutes

Vegan, gluten-free

Vegan-friendly, this burger with its delicious taste and texture packs a mighty health punch, containing folate, iron, magnesium and some omega-3 from the chia seeds. The black beans have an impressive protein profile, but these burgers are still carb dominant and therefore a great fuel choice. I love them on a bun with some salad and relish.

1 tbsp chia seeds

400g can black beans, drained and rinsed

½ tsp cayenne pepper

1 tsp ground cumin

1 tsp smoked paprika

1 tbsp tomato ketchup

2 garlic cloves, crushed, or 2 tsp garlic paste

1 onion, finely chopped

70g (¾ cup) porridge oats

a small handful of fresh coriander, leaves chopped

panko breadcrumbs, to coat (optional)

olive oil, for shallow-frying

salt and ground black pepper

1. Put the chia seeds in a small bowl and add 3 tbsp water. Set aside for 5–10 minutes to thicken. Stir the mixture to loosen it a bit – it will be very thick and gloopy.

2. Put the black beans in a bowl and roughly mash them. Add all ingredients (except the panko breadcrumbs and oil). Season with salt and pepper, and mix well to combine. You want to make sure that the chia seeds are evenly mixed through.

3. Using your hands, roll the mixture into four even-sized balls and flatten them into patties about 1.25cm thick.

4. If using panko breadcrumbs, put them on a plate and press the patties into them on both sides until well coated. Put the finished patties on a plate or baking sheet and into the fridge to firm up for 1–2 hours.

5. When ready to eat, pan-fry the burgers in a little oil for 4–5 minutes on each side or until golden. Serve.

Nutrition: Health score 4.1 High in iron, manganese and sodium

Kcal	Carbs	Sugar	Protein	Fat	Sat Fat	Fibre
209.1	24.7g	1.9g (2.1%)	10.7g	2.3g	0.3g (1.7%)	13.2g (44.1%)

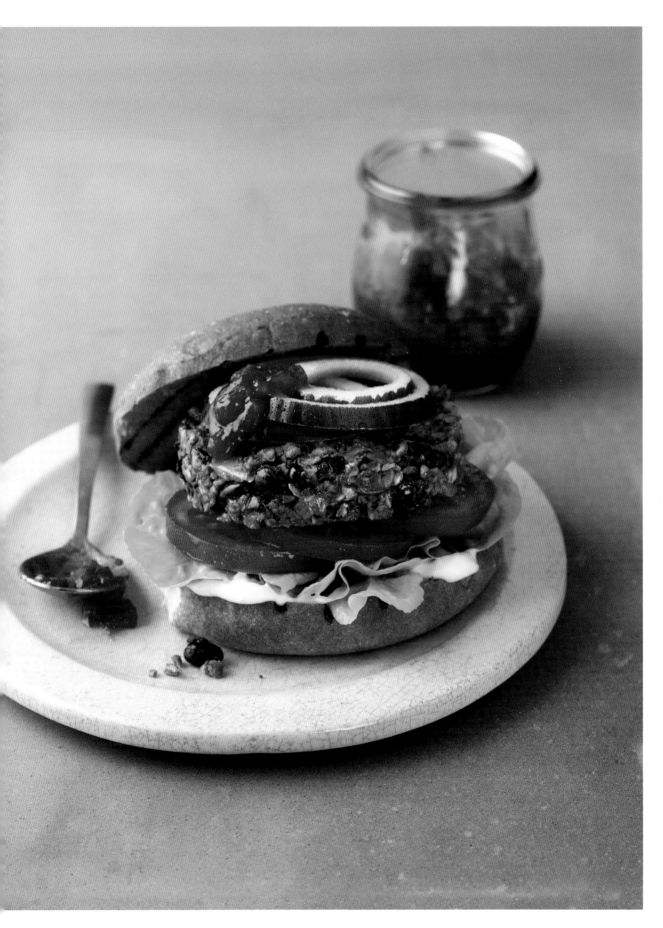

Roasted Vegetable Lasagne

Serves 4

Prep. 15 minutes

Vegetarian

You have to try this vegetarian slant on the Italian classic to believe how tasty it is, and you won't miss the meat version at all. It provides over 100 per cent of the recommended daily allowance (RDA) for vitamins A and C, and a host of phytonutrients, which are key to good health and well-being. It's Fuel dominant, but it has an impressive 18g of protein, and is therefore a great choice to eat around exercise, especially to enhance recovery.

½ onion, cut into chunks

1 red onion, cut into chunks

2 courgettes, cut into chunks

2 carrots, cut into small chunks

1 red pepper, seeded and cut into chunks

1 green pepper, seeded and cut into chunks

100g celery, chopped

olive oil spray

400g can chopped tomatoes

3 tbsp tomato purée

1 tbsp smoked paprika

1 tbsp dried oregano

2 garlic cloves, crushed, or 1 tbsp garlic paste

12 no pre-cook lasagne sheets

50g low-fat cheese, grated

salt and ground black pepper

For the béchamel sauce

50g butter

50g cornflour

500ml milk

1. Preheat the oven to 180°C (160°C fan oven) Gas 4. Put the onions, courgettes, carrots, peppers and celery into a roasting tin and spray with oil. Season with salt and pepper, and roast for 30 minutes or until golden.

2. Put the tomatoes in a saucepan over a medium-high heat and add the tomato purée, paprika, oregano and garlic. Bring to the boil, then reduce the heat and simmer for 10 minutes, or until the roasted veg are ready.

3. To make the béchamel sauce, melt the butter in a saucepan over a medium heat, then slowly add the flour, stirring gently. Gradually add the milk, stirring continuously until thickened. Season with salt and pepper.

4. Tip the roasted veg into the pan with the tomato sauce.

5. Transfer the tomato mixture to a large ovenproof dish and cover with the pasta sheets, then top with the béchamel sauce. Sprinkle over the cheese, then cook in the oven for 35 minutes or until golden. Serve.

Nutrition: Health score 8.7 High in vitamins A, C and K

Kcal	Carbs	Sugar	Protein	Fat	Sat Fat	Fibre
432.6	51.4g	16.5g (18.3%)	18.5g	13.2g	7.3g (36.7%)	8.6g (22.6%)

Slow-Cooker Butternut Squash and Lentil Curry

Serves 2

Prep. 15 minutes

Vegan, gluten-free

Slow-cooked curries are incredibly easy and hassle-free to make. For this reason I would recommend buying a slow cooker: you can pick them up quite cheaply and they use very little electricity, so they are an economical way to cook meals. You can simply put the ingredients in the slow-cooker crock and the flavours will develop while it cooks at a very low temperature all day. This dish is rich in flavour and nutrients; in fact there are too many vitamins and minerals that have a high RDA to mention here. The vegetables provide a high Health content, but you can also eat it with rice or another whole grain to make it a great Fuel choice for exercise.

350g red lentils

550g canned chopped tomatoes

400ml coconut milk

1 tsp ground turmeric

1 tsp ground cumin

1 tsp garam masala

2 vegetable stock cubes

5cm fresh ginger, peeled and grated

1 onion, chopped

1½ tbsp curry powder

2 garlic cloves, crushed, or 2 tsp garlic paste

550g peeled butternut squash, cubed

salt and ground black pepper

1 tbsp chopped fresh coriander, to garnish

Put all the ingredients (except the coriander) in a slow cooker and cook for 8 hours on low. Top with the coriander and serve.

Nutrition: Health score 18.3 High in vitamins B1, B6 and A

Kcal	Carbs	Sugar	Protein	Fat	Sat Fat	Fibre
566	73.3g	19.1g (21.2%)	27.4g	8.8g	3.8g (19%)	34.7g (115.6%)

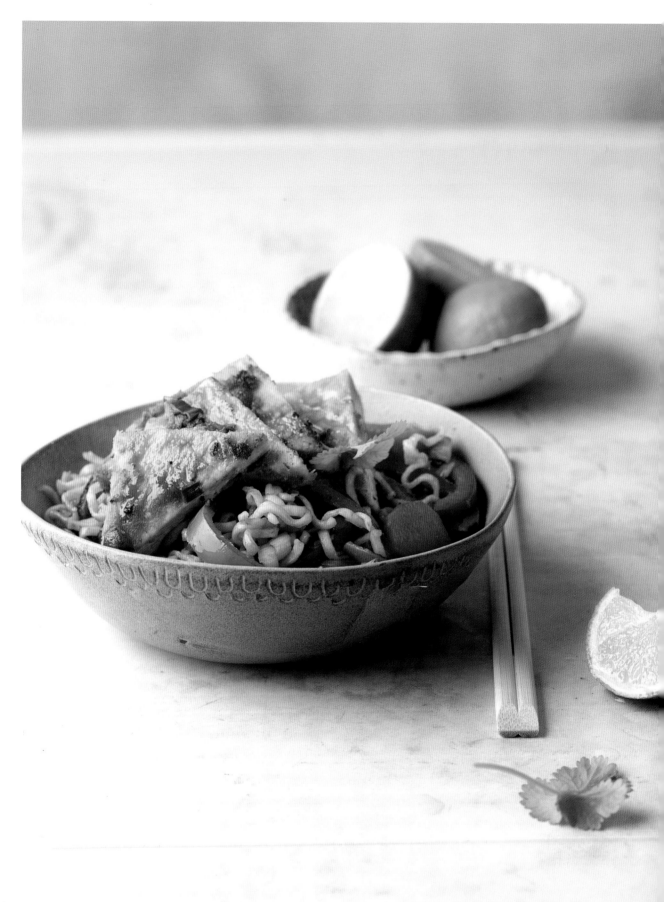

Peanut Butter Tempeh with Stir-Fry Noodles

Serves 1

Prep. 12 minutes

Vegan

This vegan-friendly stir-fry is an all-round winner. It is easy to make, packs a hefty protein punch for a vegan dish, and is a good Fuel and Health choice. Most of all it's delicious and richly flavoured with peanut butter. It has a great nutritional profile: high in B vitamins, which are good for the metabolism; vitamins A and C, which are good for eye health and immunity; and numerous minerals, such as phosphorus, iron and zinc.

125g tempeh, thawed if frozen, cut into triangles

1 tbsp peanut butter

1 tsp honey or maple syrup

2 tsp soy sauce

2 garlic cloves, crushed, or 2 tsp garlic paste

1 wholewheat noodle nest

1 tsp sesame oil

3 spring onions, sliced

½ green pepper, seeded and sliced

½ red pepper, seeded and sliced

½ carrot, very thinly sliced

coriander leaves, to garnish

ground black pepper

lime wedge, to serve

1. Put the tempeh into a bowl of warm water and soak for 5 minutes. Drain in a colander.

2. Put the peanut butter into a bowl and add the honey, 1 tsp of the soy sauce and the garlic. Add the tempeh and toss to coat, then leave to marinate while you prepare the other ingredients.

3. Boil a saucepan of water and add the noodle nest. Return to the boil, then turn off the heat and leave for 4 minutes or until tender, or according to the pack instructions. Drain in a colander.

4. Heat ½ tsp sesame oil in a frying pan or wok over a medium-high heat and add the vegetables. Cook for 3 minutes.

5. Add the tempeh and cook for a further 5 minutes, turning regularly.

6. Stir the cooked vegetables into the noodles and add ½ tsp sesame oil and 1 tsp soy sauce. Garnish with coriander leaves and black pepper, and serve with a lime wedge.

Nutrition: Health score 12.6 High in vitamins B6, A and C

Kcal	Carbs	Sugar	Protein	Fat	Sat Fat	Fibre
696.4	70.2g	21g (22.3%)	41.5g	28g	5.8g (29.1%)	15.3g (50.9%)

Vegan Sausages

Serves 4

Prep. 10 minutes

Vegan, gluten-free

These vegan sausages have a meaty taste and texture and are made without additives, which are commonly used in bought vegan sausages. The bean and veggies make them Fuel based, but there is plenty of protein and, obviously, Health, with vitamins A and C above 25 per cent of the RDA. They are so easy to make – you'd be bangers not to try them!

3 sweet potatoes, diced

2 tsp olive oil, plus extra to drizzle

400g can kidney beans, drained and rinsed

1 tbsp tomato purée

1 tsp dried oregano

1 tsp paprika

1 tsp tamari or soy sauce

1. Preheat the oven to 190°C (170°C fan oven) Gas 5. Put the sweet potatoes in a roasting tin and drizzle with a little olive oil, then roast for 15 minutes or until soft.

2. Put the kidney beans and the roasted sweet potatoes in a bowl and lightly mash together to a semi-purée.

3. Add the remaining ingredients, (except the olive oil), and mix until well combined.

4. Roll the mixture into sausage shapes using your hands.

5. Heat the 2 tsp olive oil in a frying pan over a medium-low heat and fry the sausages, turning occasionally, for 5–8 minutes or until browned on all sides. Serve.

Nutrition: Health score 8 High in vitamins B6, D and selenium

Kcal	Carbs	Sugar	Protein	Fat	Sat Fat	Fibre
226.7	31.6g	9.8g (10.8%)	10.1g	3.5g	0.6g (2.8%)	8.8g (29.2%)

Spicy Prawns with Quinoa

Serves 2

Prep. 15 minutes

When I want a balanced meal with little preparation to make quickly during the week, I often go for this simple but tasty Spanish-inspired meal. Quinoa now comes in handy quick- cook packets and is a good carb choice because it has a relatively low glycaemic index (see page 221) for a grain and contains all the essential amino acids. Prawns are a lean protein option and peas contain a good amount of vitamin C. The spices and garlic are anti-inflammatory as well as giving the dish its zing.

1 tsp and 1 tbsp olive oil

½ onion, finely chopped

200ml vegetable stock

125g frozen peas

225g raw or cooked shelled prawns

2 garlic cloves, crushed, or 2 tsp garlic paste

1–2 tsp chilli powder, to taste

200g ready-to-eat quinoa

salt and ground black pepper

1. Heat the 1 teaspoon of oil in a saucepan over a medium heat, add the onion and cook for 3 minutes.

2. Add the stock and peas, bring to the boil, then reduce the heat and simmer for 8 minutes.

3. Meanwhile, heat the 1 tbsp oil in another pan. Add the prawns, garlic and chilli powder and cook the until the prawns are pink.

4. Microwave the quinoa according to the pack instructions.

5. Add the quinoa and prawns to the stock and simmer for 1–2 minutes until heated through and blended. Season to taste and serve.

Nutrition: Health score 7.2 High in vitamins A, B12 and copper

Kcal	Carbs	Sugar	Protein	Fat	Sat Fat	Fibre
352.3	31.1g	6.4g (7.1%)	39.1g	5.2g	0.8g (3.8%)	7.8g (26%)

Salmon, Tomato and Asparagus Bake

Serves 2

Prep. 10 minutes

Gluten-free

A Mediterranean-inspired dish that is light, easy to make and full of flavour. Salmon provides an excellent source of protein and omega-3 fatty acids, while the soy marinade contains a class of phytochemicals called isoflavones, which help to promote a healthy heart. Asparagus and tomatoes are rich in various vitamins and minerals. New potatoes have a lower glycaemic index than older potatoes, helping to keep blood sugar stable.

8 new potatoes, halved

4 tomatoes, halved

200g asparagus spears, tough ends removed

4 individual salmon fillets

1 lemon, halved

olive oil, to drizzle

1 tbsp tamari or soy sauce

2 tbsp balsamic vinegar

1. Preheat the oven to 200°C (180°C fan oven) Gas 6.

2. Part-cook the potatoes in a saucepan of boiling water for 10 minutes. Drain in a colander.

3. Put the tomatoes, asparagus and salmon, skin-side up, in a roasting tin.

4. Add the potatoes to the tin. Squeeze the lemon juice over the fish and vegetables.

5. Drizzle a little olive oil over everything, then sprinkle over the soy sauce and balsamic. Cook in the oven for 18–20 minutes. Serve.

Nutrition: Health score 14 High in vitamins A, C and K

Kcal	Carbs	Sugar	Protein	Fat	Sat Fat	Fibre
656.9	45.6g	12.9g (14.3%)	57.7g	18.3g	2.8g (14%)	10.9g (36.3%)

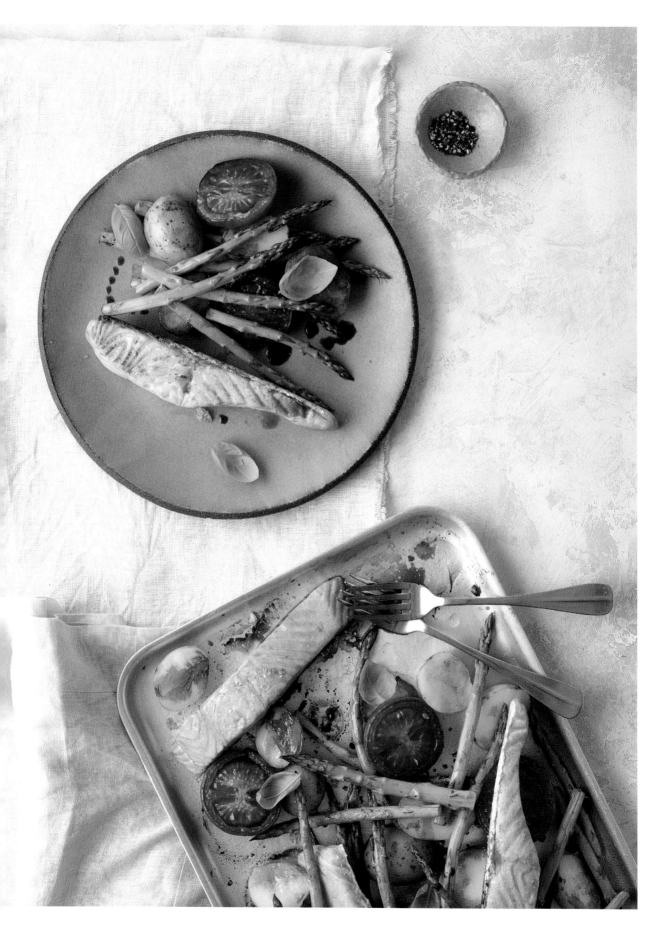

Hake with Sautéed Vegetables

Serves 2
—
Prep. 7 minutes
—
Gluten-free
—

Impress your friends and family with this classy-looking disk, which is actually surprisingly simple to make. Hake is a lovely meaty fish with great texture. The various vegetables provide vitamins and minerals important for healthy eyes, bones and skin. This is a low-carb, low-calorie dish that is ideal for weight loss.

2 tbsp olive oil

2 individual hake fillets, with skin

½ onion, sliced

100g mushrooms, sliced

8 cherry tomatoes, halved

2 large handfuls of baby spinach

salt and ground black pepper

1. Heat 1 tbsp oil in a frying pan over a medium heat and pan-fry the hake, skin-side first for 4–5 minutes until golden, then flip the hake over and cook for a further 4–5 minutes until golden. Preheat the grill.

2. Heat 1 tbsp oil in a frying pan over a medium heat and cook the onion and mushrooms for 5 minutes or until golden. Add the tomatoes and spinach, and season with salt and pepper to taste, and stir through briefly. Remove from the heat.

3. Put the hake under the grill for 3–4 minutes until cooked through and the flesh separates easily with a knife. Serve the hake with the vegetables on top.

Nutrition: Health score 7.7 High in vitamins A, C and K

Kcal	Carbs	Sugar	Protein	Fat	Sat Fat	Fibre
150	5.6g	4.1g (4.5%)	24.5g	2.5g	0.5g (2.6%)	2.4g (6.3%)

Smoked Haddock Kedgeree

Serves 2

Prep. 16 minutes

My version of this traditional dish is easy to make and provides a balanced meal with bags of flavour. Haddock contains some omega-3 fats and, with the eggs, provides a good dose of protein. Healthy onions and peas combine with a convenient carb source of quick-cook rice to make a speedy, fuss-free meal. Kedgeree is a good choice leading up to exertive exercise without carrying a high calorie load.

2 eggs

1 tsp olive oil

2 tbsp masala curry paste

¼ onion, finely chopped

1 smoked haddock fillet, flaked into small chunks

1 packet microwave vegetable rice

70g frozen peas

1. Put the eggs in a saucepan of boiling water. Return to the boil and cook for 10 minutes. Drain the pan and refill with cold water. Drain and fill again. Leave the eggs to cool, then peel off the shells. Set aside.

2. Heat the oil in large saucepan over a medium heat. Add the curry paste, onion and haddock, and cook for 5 minutes.

3. Meanwhile, cook the vegetable rice for 2 minutes, or according to the pack instructions.

4. Tip the rice into the pan with the haddock mixture and add the peas, then cook for 4 minutes.

5. Slice the boiled eggs. Serve the kedgeree with the eggs on top.

Nutrition: Health score 4.6 High in vitamin A, iron and selenium

Kcal	Carbs	Sugar	Protein	Fat	Sat Fat	Fibre
276.5	31.1g	3.8g (4.2%)	16.8g	7.8g	2.3g (11.3%)	2.5g (8.4%)

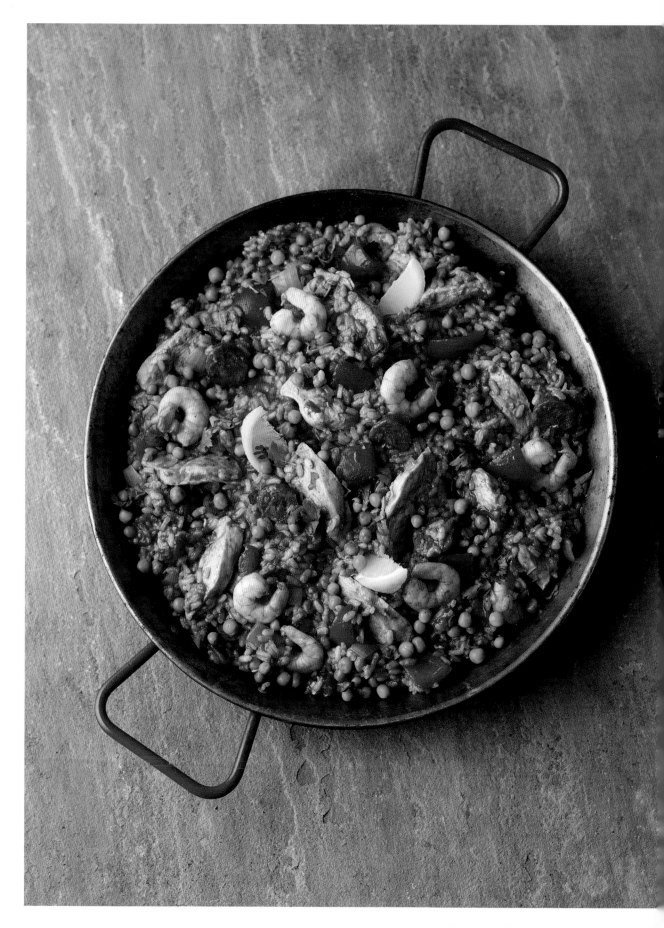

Power Paella

Serves 4

Prep. 25 minutes

A Spanish classic that packs a big flavour punch, paella is right up there in my favourite meals. It provides a good portion of carbs and protein, and is therefore ideal to aid recovery after exertive exercise. This recipe provides a range of B vitamins, which are important for energy production, in addition to numerous minerals.

1 tbsp olive oil

4 skinless chicken breasts, sliced

1 large onion, chopped

2 garlic cloves, crushed, or 2 tsp garlic paste

100g chorizo, skinned and sliced

1 red pepper, seeded and chopped

1 tbsp paprika

1 tsp ground turmeric

700ml chicken stock

400g can chopped tomatoes

280g paella rice

200g frozen peas

100g raw or cooked shelled prawns

salt and ground black pepper

1. Heat the oil in a large frying pan. Add the chicken, onion and garlic, and cook for 10 minutes or until the chicken is white, turning regularly.

2. Add the chorizo, pepper, paprika and turmeric, and fry for 2 minutes.

3. Add the chicken stock and tomatoes, then season with salt and pepper. Bring to the boil, add the rice and stir well. Return to the boil, then reduce the heat and simmer very gently for 20 minutes.

4. Stir in the peas and prawns, and cook for 5 minutes until the prawns are pink and cooked through.

5. The paella is cooked when it has absorbed most of the water, leaving the rice moist; stir only occasionally to stop the rice from sticking to the base of the pan. Serve.

Nutrition: Health score 7 High in vitamins B3, B6 and A

Kcal	Carbs	Sugar	Protein	Fat	Sat Fat	Fibre
517.3	33.3g	11g (12.3%)	52.1g	15.9g	5.4g (27%)	6.4g (21.3%)

Fish Pie

Serves 2

Prep. 15 minutes

Gluten-free

People are often intimidated by making a fish pie, because it seems complicated, but I promise you that this version is easy to prepare. It provides a really good dose of carbs and protein, and so it is a great choice to eat after training or when being very active. The fish provides a lean protein source and, if salmon is used, omega-3 fats, which are anti-inflammatory and good for a healthy heart and brain. Spring onions, peas and spinach are immunity boosters, and the potato mash provides carbs, and works with the sauce to give the dish a lovely creamy texture.

500ml semi-skimmed milk, plus extra for the potatoes

600g diced fish-pie mix, or cod, haddock or salmon, cut into cubes

3 tbsp cornflour

1 tsp English mustard

100g frozen peas

6 spring onions, chopped

1 tbsp chopped fresh dill

1 large handful baby spinach

300g potatoes, peeled and cut into large chunks

salt and ground black pepper

1. Pour the milk into a saucepan over a medium heat and bring to a gentle simmer. Add the fish and gently poach for 5 minutes or until cooked through. Drain in a colander, saving the milk.

2. Put the milk back into the pan over a medium-low heat. Put the cornflour in a small bowl and gradually stir in 4 tbsp water until smooth and creamy. Gradually add this to the milk, whisking continuously until thickened.

3. Add the mustard, peas, spring onions, dill and spinach to the sauce. Season with salt and pepper, and mix well.

4. Put a layer of the sauce mixture into a pie dish, then cover with the fish. Top with the remaining sauce mixture. Leave to cool.

5. Meanwhile, preheat the oven to 190°C (170°C fan oven) Gas 5. Cook the potatoes in a saucepan of boiling water for 15 minutes or until tender. Drain in a colander, then return them to the pan.

6. Add a splash of milk to the potatoes and season with salt and pepper. Mash them until creamy. Top the fish filling with the mash, smoothing it evenly up to the edge of the dish. Cook in the oven for 30–40 minutes until golden brown. Serve.

Nutrition: Health score 12.5 High in vitamins B6, B12 and A

Kcal	Carbs	Sugar	Protein	Fat	Sat Fat	Fibre
720.8	63.6g	17.4g (19.3%)	85.4g	9g	3.6g (17.9%)	9.7g (32.5%)

Lemon Sea Bass and Asparagus Bake

Serves 1

Prep. 6 minutes

Gluten-free

You have to try this zesty lemon sea bass dish that you can make with minimal fuss. The dish is low-calorie and high-protein, making it suitable for those who want to be lean or who are having a low-activity day. The asparagus accompaniment also offers some serious health benefits, containing an array of micronutrients and powerful antioxidants to reduce cell damage.

1 tbsp lemon juice

1 tbsp tamari or soy sauce

a pinch of dried chilli flakes

1 sea bass fillet

5 asparagus spears, tough ends removed

1 lemon, sliced

1. Preheat the oven to 200°C (180°C fan oven) Gas 6.

2. Pour the lemon juice into a bowl and add the soy sauce and chilli flakes. Mix until combined.

3. Put the sea bass and asparagus on a baking sheet. Put the lemon slices evenly over the top, then spoon over the sauce. Cook in the oven for 15–20 minutes or until the fish is cooked through and the flesh separates easily with a knife. Serve.

Nutrition: Health score 5.3 High in vitamins B6, D and selenium

Kcal	Carbs	Sugar	Protein	Fat	Sat Fat	Fibre
169.3	5.4g	2.3g (2.6%)	28.5g	3.1g	0.8g (3.8%)	2.8g (9.3%)

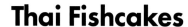

Thai Fishcakes

Serves 2

Prep. 15 minutes

Gluten-free

Spice up your fishcakes with Thai flavourings. These cod fishcakes provide a high-protein, low-carbohydrate alternative to traditional potato-based fishcakes, so they are perfect for anyone trying to lose weight. And they taste great! Cod also provides a moderate amount of omega-3 fats which helps to reduce inflammation and may also help with muscle building by increasing our sensitivity to the amino acids in the fish.

250g cod fillet, bones removed

1 red chilli, seeded

2 tsp lemongrass paste

2 spring onions, finely chopped

2 tbsp roughly chopped coriander

2 tsp fish sauce

1 egg

2 tbsp desiccated coconut

1 tbsp coconut oil (or other cooking oil)

1 lime, sliced, to serve (optional)

1. Put the cod, chilli, lemongrass paste, spring onions, coriander, fish sauce, egg and desiccated coconut into a food processor. Pulse until the ingredients form a paste.

2. Shape the mixture into patties as desired (I recommend about 3–4cm thick).

3. Heat the oil in frying pan and fry the fishcakes for 3 minutes on each side or until golden and cooked through. Serve with a slice of lime if you like.

Nutrition: Health score 8.9 High in vitamins A, B6 and B12

Kcal	Carbs	Sugar	Protein	Fat	Sat Fat	Fibre
388.7	10.5g	9.6g (10.6%)	49.3g	15g	5.8g (28.8%)	2.6g (8.6%)

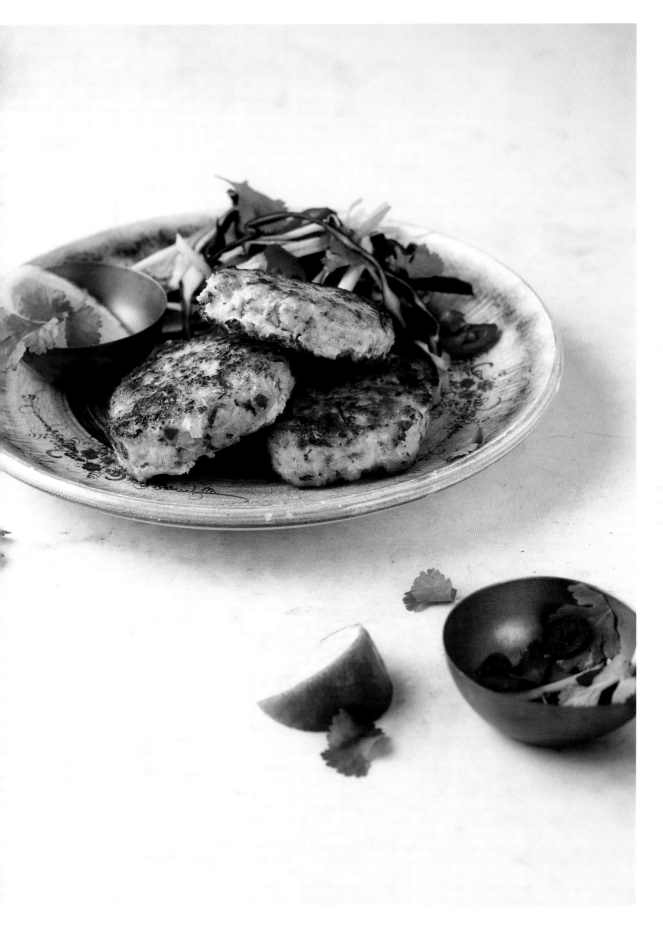

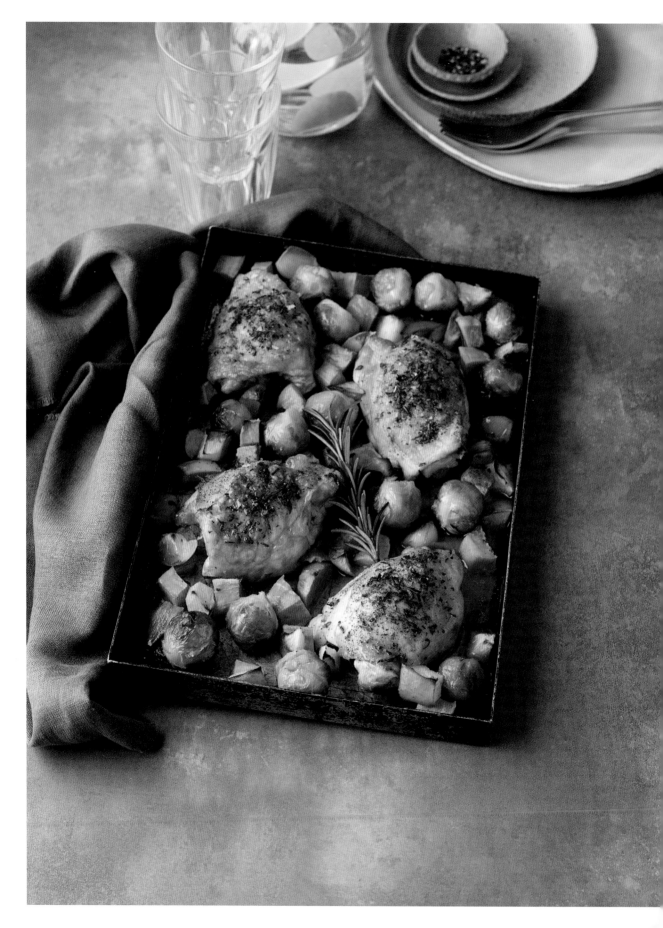

Autumn Chicken and Veggie Bake

Serves 2

Prep. 10 minutes

Gluten-free

This one-tray bake is mega-easy to make. It reflects autumn through its dark orange and green colours and welcoming flavours of rosemary and thyme. It is a nicely balanced meal suitable for most occasions, and it is high in several vitamins and minerals, especially B vitamins, which are important for energy metabolism.

4 skin-on chicken thighs

1 tbsp fresh chopped rosemary

1 tbsp fresh thyme

1 sweet potato, cut into small chunks

400g Brussels sprouts

2 dessert apples, cut into chunks

3 garlic cloves, peeled and left whole

1 tbsp olive oil

salt and ground black pepper

1. Preheat the oven to 220°C (200°C fan oven) Gas 7. Season the chicken thighs with the rosemary, thyme, salt and pepper.

2. Put all the ingredients in a roasting tin and drizzle with the olive oil. Season.

3. Bake for 30–35 minutes until the chicken thighs are cooked through and the juices are clear. Serve.

Nutrition: Health score 16.6 High in vitamins B6, A and C

Kcal	Carbs	Sugar	Protein	Fat	Sat Fat	Fibre
532.4	43.1g	27.1g (30.1%)	44.9g	16g	3.7g (18.3%)	15.1g (50.5%)

Chicken Biriyani

Serves 3

Prep. 12 minutes

Biriyani is a mixed rice dish that originates from India. It is a richly flavoured and well-balanced meal that is wonderfully spicy. The rice makes it Fuel dominant, but there is lots of Lean Muscle and Health too. The various spices are anti-inflammatory and the tomatoes and peppers provide plenty of vitamin C to support immunity. The chicken breasts are cooked in the oven for ease, but if you prefer you can chop them and add with the garlic and spices.

2 chicken breasts

300g brown basmati rice

2 tbsp olive oil

2 red onions, chopped

2 garlic cloves, crushed, or 2 tsp garlic paste

2.5cm fresh ginger, finely chopped

1 tsp ground cardamom

1 tsp ground coriander

½ tsp ground cinnamon

½ tsp ground turmeric

1 tsp dried chilli flakes

500ml chicken stock

juice of 1 lime

1. Preheat the oven to 200°C (180°C fan oven) Gas 6. Loosely wrap the chicken breasts in foil, place on a baking tray and cook for approximately 25 minutes (a little less if the breasts are small).

2. Heat the olive oil in a saucepan over a medium heat, add the onions and cook for 5 minutes or until they are translucent. Add the garlic, ginger, cardamom, coriander, cinnamon, turmeric and chilli flakes. Mix together and cook for a further 2 minutes.

3. Pour the chicken stock into the pan. Add the rice to the pan, cover with a lid and simmer for 20–25 minutes until the rice is tender.

4. Remove the chicken from the oven, chop into small chunks and add to the rice. Add the lime juice to the pan, mix through and cook for a further 2 minutes. Serve.

Nutrition: Health score 8.3 High in vitamins B3, B6 and C

Kcal	Carbs	Sugar	Protein	Fat	Sat Fat	Fibre
539.6	44.7g	11.9g (13.2%)	35.5g	22g	5g (25.1%)	7.3g (24.9%)

Chicken and Mushroom Risotto

Serves 1

Prep. 15 minutes

Risottos are rich and delicious, and this version is no exception. It packs a big carb and protein punch and so it is a great choice for fuelling and recovery. Mushrooms contain various nutrients, including B vitamins, selenium, potassium and copper, which are important for energy production and immune function.

100g risotto rice

1 tbsp olive oil

6 mushrooms, chopped

⅓ leek, white part only, chopped

1 large chicken breast, cut into cubes

juice of 1 lemon

250ml chicken stock

salt and ground black pepper

1. Bring a large saucepan of water to the boil, and boil the rice for 5 minutes. Drain in a colander.

2. Heat the oil in a saucepan over a medium heat and add the mushrooms, leek and chicken. Fry for 2 minutes.

3. Add the rice to the pan and fry with the other ingredients for 1 minute. Add the chicken stock to the pan and simmer for 10-12 minutes until the chicken and rice are cooked. Serve.

Nutrition: Health score 5.1 High in vitamins B2, A and C

Kcal	Carbs	Sugar	Protein	Fat	Sat Fat	Fibre
671	79g	5.9g (6.6%)	68g	7.8g	6g (30%)	2.4g (7.6%)

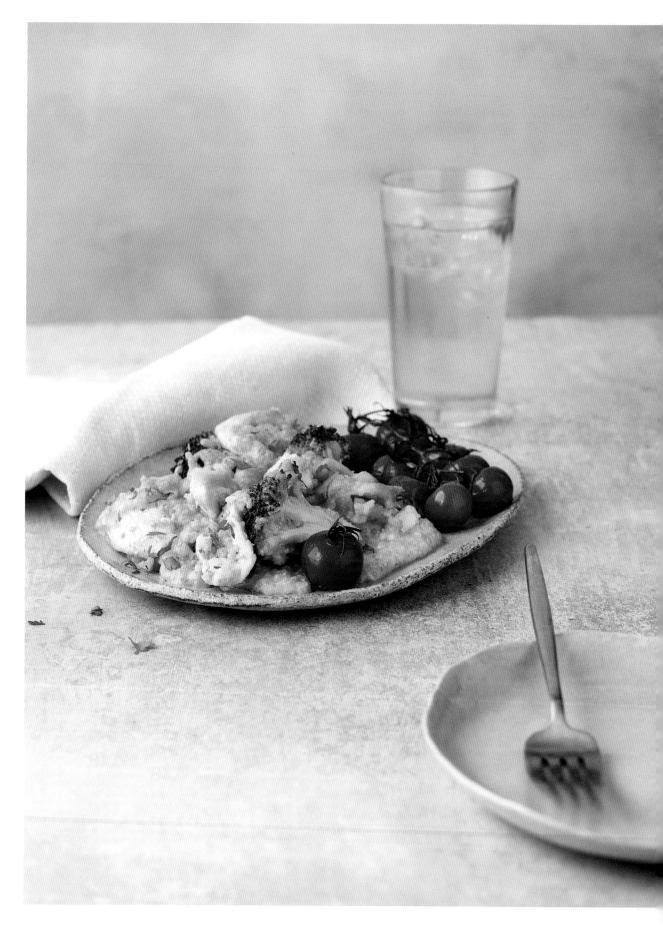

Creamy Chicken, Quinoa and Broccoli Bake

Serves 3

Prep. 15 minutes

Although 'creamy' is not synonymous with health, we have made this satisfising dinner as healthy as possible by eliminating the cream and minimising the butter, while maximising taste. It is a delicious all-round meal – the chicken provides a lean source of protein, quinoa is a relatively low-glycaemic carb (see page 221) that has a complete amino acid profile, and broccoli is a wonder vegetable, rich fibre and in antioxidants that help fight disease.

425ml stock made with ½ chicken stock cube and ½ vegetable stock cube

250ml semi-skimmed milk

2 cloves garlic, chopped or 1 tsp garlic paste

1 tsp dried thyme

1 head of broccoli, cut into florets

25g unsalted butter

70g (½ cup) flour

3 chicken breasts, cut into thin strips

200g pre-cooked quinoa

40g Parmesan or Cheddar cheese, grated

1. Preheat the oven to 200°C (180°C fan oven) Gas 6.
2. Pour the stock and milk into a saucepan, add the garlic and thyme and simmer over a medium heat for 5 minutes.
3. Boil or steam the broccoli for 4–5 minutes, then leave to drain.
4. Meanwhile, place another pan over a medium heat, than add the butter to melt. Add the flour, then add a little of the stock, stirring constantly to make a paste. Slowly add the remaining stock, mixing constantly for 3–4 minutes until smooth and creamy. If the mix remains lumpy, use a whisk to break it up.
5. Spread the chicken and quinoa over an ovenproof dish. Pour over the sauce and mix well. Cook in the oven for 20 minutes, then remove and add the broccoli, mix through and cover with the grated cheese.
6. Return to the oven and cook for a further 10 minutes. Serve.

Nutrition: Health score 9.4 High in vitamins B3, B6 and C

Kcal	Carbs	Sugar	Protein	Fat	Sat Fat	Fibre
590	37.4g	6.7g (7.5%)	55.6g	21.5g	9.7g (48.6%)	6.9g (22.9%)

Turkey Bolognese

Serves 2

Prep. 10 minutes

Using turkey instead of the traditional beef for this twist on an Italian classic makes the dish leaner due to its reduced fat content. The delicious sauce makes it just as tasty though. This meal provides a good amount of both carbs and protein making it the perfect food for recovery after hard training days.

500g minced turkey

½ red onion, chopped

1 carrot, chopped

1 celery stick, chopped

200g can chopped tomatoes

3 garlic cloves, crushed, or 3 tsp garlic paste

2 tbsp tomato purée

1 tbsp dried oregano

200g wholemeal pasta

salt and ground black pepper

spinach, to serve

1. Put the turkey in a saucepan over a medium heat and add the onion, carrot and celery. Cook for 5 minutes until the mince is sealed – use a whisk to break up the mince.

2. Add the tomatoes, garlic, tomato purée and oregano, and season with salt and pepper. Bring to the boil.

3. Reduce the heat and simmer for 20 minutes, stirring occasionally, until the tomatoes have broken down and the sauce begins to thicken.

4. Meanwhile, cook the pasta in a saucepan of boiling water for 8–10 minutes until tender with a bite, or according to the pack instructions. Serve the bolognese with the pasta and spinach.

Nutrition: Health score 3.3 High in vitamin A and sodium

Kcal	Carbs	Sugar	Protein	Fat	Sat Fat	Fibre
730.9	77.6g	10.7g (11.9%)	63.3g	14.8g	4.4g (22%)	12.2g (40.7%)

Healthy Chicken Pie

Serves 4

Prep. 18 minutes

If you think that cooking a pie is complicated and time-consuming, this recipe will smash that myth – with the added bonus that it is healthy and tasty. The crème fraîche makes a creamy sauce that is lower in saturated fat than using cream. Chicken is a lean protein, and leeks are part of the onion family, which contain the anti-inflammatory compound allicin.

1 tbsp olive oil

4 large skinless chicken breasts, diced

2 leeks, sliced

40g button mushrooms, sliced

1 tbsp flour

300ml low-fat crème fraîche

150ml chicken stock

1 tbsp English mustard

1 tsp freshly grated nutmeg

1 sheet of ready-rolled puff pastry

1 egg, beaten

salt and ground black pepper

1. Heat the oil in a large frying pan over a medium-high heat and cook the chicken for 10 minutes or until white.

2. Add the leeks and mushrooms, and cook for 2 minutes. Sprinkle the flour over the mixture and stir for 1 minute using a wooden spoon. Stir in the crème fraîche and the stock, mustard and nutmeg until creamy. Bring back to the boil, and season with salt and pepper. Transfer to an ovenproof dish.

3. Meanwhile preheat the oven to 200°C (180°C fan oven) Gas 6. Unroll the pastry and put it over the top of the pie, pushing down the edges. Brush the pastry with beaten egg. Cook in the oven for 15 minutes or until golden brown. Serve.

Nutrition: Health score 3.5 High in vitamins B3, B6 and selenium

Kcal	Carbs	Sugar	Protein	Fat	Sat Fat	Fibre
347.5	8.7g	3.1g (3.5%)	40.7g	15.5g	6.5g (32.9%)	1.3g (4.2%)

Rapid Chicken Sunday Dinner

Serves 1

Prep. 15 minutes

Gluten-free

A Sunday roast without all the fuss – what could be better? Ready in under 30 minutes, this quick-fix chicken roast is the perfect way to recover from a hard week of training. It provides a balanced combination of protein and carbohydrate to repair and replenish, but that's not all: it's health benefits are quite staggering, with one of the highest health scores in Colour-Fit.

1 large sweet potato, cut into 8 wedges

olive oil, for drizzling

1 chicken breast, or vegan alternative

gravy mix to make 200ml gravy, or vegan alternative

100g broccoli, cut into florets

1 carrot, thinly sliced

50g kale, stalks removed

50g mangetout

salt and ground black pepper

1. Preheat the oven to 210°C (190°C fan oven) Gas 6½. Put the sweet potato wedges in a roasting tin and sprinkle with salt, pepper and olive oil. Roast for 20–30 minutes until golden.

2. Meanwhile, slice horizontally through 80 per cent of the chicken breast and open it out to make a butterfly. Season with salt, pepper and a light drizzle of olive oil.

3. Preheat a griddle pan over a medium-high heat and cook the chicken for 5 minutes on each side or until golden and cooked through and the juices run clear. Make the gravy according to the pack instructions while the chicken is cooking.

4. Bring a saucepan of boiling water to a rolling boil and cook the carrot and broccoli for 3 minutes. Add the kale and mangetout and cook for 30 seconds or until cooked but still bright green. Drain in a colander. Serve the chicken with the sweet potato wedges, vegetables and gravy.

Nutrition: Health Score 13.9 High in vitamins B1, B5, A, copper and iron

Kcal	Curbs	Sugar	Protein	Fat	Sat Fat	Fibre
515.7	50.5g	22g (24.5%)	48.2g	8.5g	2.2g (11%)	13.1g (34.6%)

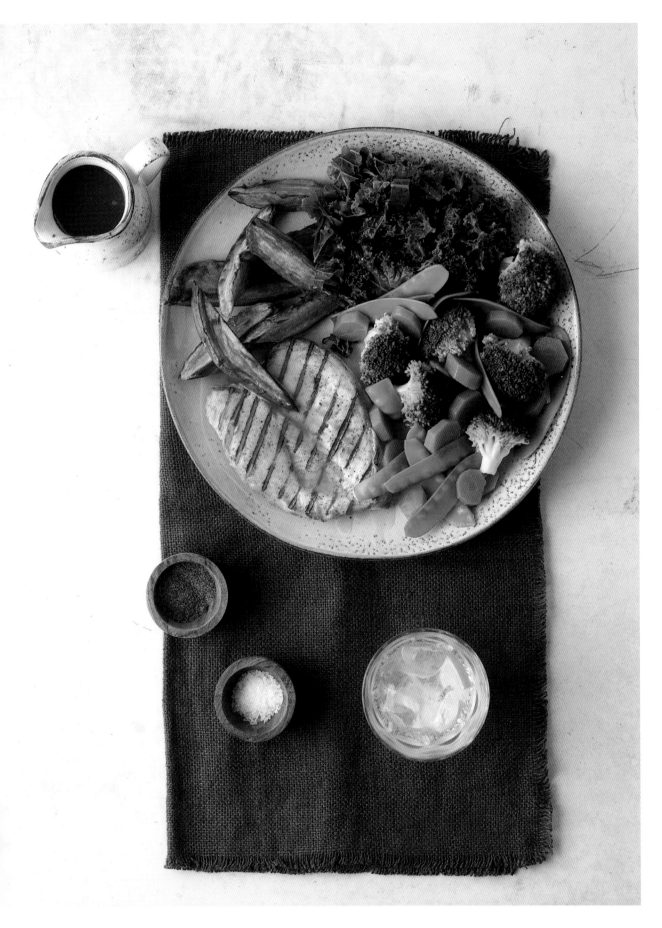

Turkey Burgers with Feta and Spinach

Serves 2

Prep. 16 minutes

Gluten-free

My turkey burgers provide the perfect hit of protein without the guilt that might come with traditional burgers. Protein is important to kick-start the muscle remodelling process, so these burgers are a great choice to eat after any resistance training. They can be combined with a bun to provide carbohydrate, making this meal a winning combination for recovery. The feta, which is a low-fat cheese, adds bags of flavour and texture, and spinach adds a hit of antioxidants and nitrates, which can aid recovery.

2 large handfuls of baby spinach

400g minced turkey

1–2 garlic cloves, to taste, crushed, or 1–2 tsp garlic paste

1 egg, beaten

60g feta cheese, crumbled

olive oil, if needed

salt and ground black pepper

bread buns, onion and tomato to serve (optional)

1. Put the spinach in a saucepan with only the water left on the leaves after washing. Cook briefly over a medium heat until wilted. Drain in a colander.

2. Tip into a mixing bowl and add the turkey, garlic, egg and feta. Season with salt and pepper, and mix together well, using your hands.

3. Shape into two burgers 2–3cm thick.

4. Preheat the grill and cook for 5–6 minutes on each side or until the meat has browned and is cooked through. (Alternatively, fry in a lightly oiled frying pan over a medium-high heat.) Serve in buns with onion and tomato, if you like.

Nutrition: Health score 3.1 High in vitamins A, K and protein

Kcal	Carbs	Sugar	Protein	Fat	Sat Fat	Fibre
288.2	4.4g	2.1g (2.3%)	35.2g	14g	6g (30.1%)	0.5g (1.2%)

Chilli Con Carne

Serves 3

Prep. 10 minutes

Gluten-free

Here is a Colour-Fit take on a classic dish. Because it is so simple and tasty, it is a regular go-to when we're stuck for ideas and in a rush for dinner. I use minced turkey here as opposed to beef or lamb to reduce the saturated fat content. The tomatoes, onion, mushrooms and beans add a variety of healthy nutrients as well as a rich flavour. It is a well-balanced dish that is suited to recovery/muscle building. If you want to increase the Fuel content, serve the chilli with rice.

1 tbsp olive oil

1 large onion, chopped

450g minced turkey

400g can chopped tomatoes

2 x 400g cans kidney beans, drained and rinsed

50g button mushrooms, halved

1 beef stock cube

1 packet chilli con carne mix

1. Heat the oil in a saucepan over a medium heat and cook the onion for 5 minutes or until softened.

2. Add the turkey and cook until browned. Add the tomatoes, beans and mushrooms, and stir well.

3. Crumble in the stock cube and add the packet of chilli mix, then stir well. Bring to the boil, then reduce the heat and simmer for 20 minutes. Serve.

Nutrition: Health score 4.7 High in iron, manganese and sodium

Kcal	Carbs	Sugar	Protein	Fat	Sat Fat	Fibre
476.3	43g	13.9g (15.4%)	39.8g	11.2g	2.6g (12.8%)	14.3g (47.8%)

Beef-Stuffed Peppers

Serves 2

Prep. 10 minutes

Gluten-free

These protein-packed stuffed peppers are something out of the ordinary and so easy to make. High in protein, low in carbs and with moderate calories, they are a good choice for those wishing to stay lean. The pepper provides Vitamins A, C and K to support a healthy immune and skeletal system and the vitamin C in the peppers will also help your body to absorb the iron from the beef. Swap the beef for turkey mince if you want to drop the calories even more.

2 red or yellow peppers

200g lean beef mince

2 garlic cloves, crushed, or 2 tsp garlic paste

2 tsp paprika

1 tbsp olive oil

20g low-fat Cheddar, grated

salt and ground black pepper

1. Preheat the oven to 190°C (170°C fan oven) Gas 5. Chop the tops off the peppers and remove the seeds.

2. Place the mince in a bowl and add the garlic, paprika and seasoning and mix through with your hands.

3. Heat the oil in a saucepan over a medium heat, add the mince and cook for approximately 5 minutes until the meat is browned.

4. Spoon the mince into the hollow peppers and then sprinkle on the cheese. Cook in the oven for 10 minutes. Alternatively, place on a microwavable plate and cook for 3½ minutes. Serve.

Nutrition: Health score 4.6 High in vitamins A, B6, C, iron

Kcal	Carbs	Sugar	Protein	Fat	Sat Fat	Fibre
239	9g	7.7g (8.6%)	35.6g	6.2g	2.7g (13.4%)	4.8g (16%)

Beef Stroganoff

Serves 2

Prep. 10 minutes

Gluten-free

This classic is a favourite in my house using Greek yogurt instead of cream for a healthy alternative. It's simple to prepare and full of flavour. The beef is a good source of iron and the onion, peppers and mushrooms provide varied health benefits. Offering a good dose of carbs and protein, this is a great choice to enjoy after training to replenish muscle glycogen and repair/build muscle.

cooking oil spray

300g lean beef frying steak, cut into strips

½ red onion, chopped

1 red pepper, cut into strips

100g mushrooms, sliced

2 tbsp smoked paprika

1 garlic clove, crushed, or 1 tsp garlic paste

1 beef stock cube

100g low-fat Greek yogurt

salt and ground black pepper

brown rice, to serve

1. Heat a frying pan with a spray of oil over a medium-high heat and fry the steak on both sides until sealed.

2. Add the onion, pepper, mushrooms, smoked paprika and garlic. Season with salt and pepper and stir to combine.

3. Dissolve the stock cube in a jug with 500ml hot water and pour onto the beef mixture.

4. Bring to the boil, then reduce the heat and simmer until the sauce is reduced by half. Remove from the heat and stir in the yogurt. Serve with brown rice.

Nutrition: Health score 4.5 High in vitamins A, C and sodium

Kcal	Carbs	Sugar	Protein	Fat	Sat Fat	Fibre
701.2	74g	9.9g (11%)	70g	10.1g	4.2g (21%)	10.7g (35.7%)

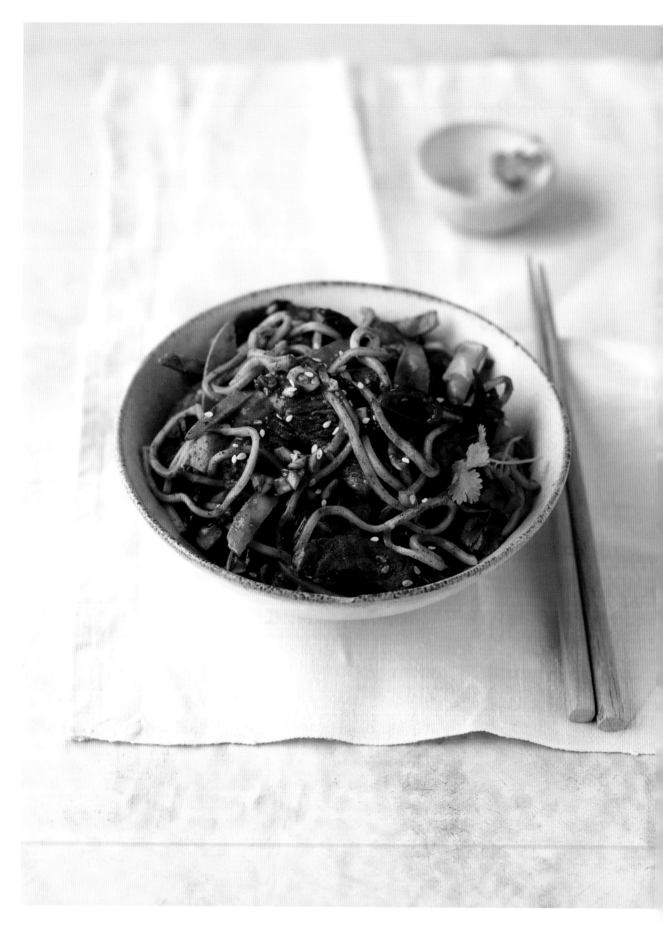

Chinese Beef Noodles

Serves 2

Prep. 15 minutes

The usual favourite from the Chinese takeaway is not a healthy choice, but speed is often the deciding factor. My version, however, is supremely tasty, and it's much better for you, plus it's ready in no time – from the comfort of your own home. Beef is a great source of B vitamins and iron in a form that is more bioavailable than plant options, red onion adds texture, taste and anti-inflammatory properties, and mangetout are high in folate and potassium. (You can use a black bean ready-made sauce if you prefer to make it even simpler.)

1 tbsp sesame oil

400g stir-fry beef strips or frying steak, cut into thin strips

2 tsp Chinese five-spice powder

1 red chilli, seeded and chopped

1 red onion, sliced

1 tbsp honey

1 garlic clove, crushed, or 1 tsp garlic paste

2 tsp peanut butter

4 tsp light soy sauce

1 tsp sesame seeds

150g mangetout, cut in half

2 packets of pre-cooked egg noodles

a handful of fresh coriander, leaves chopped

1. Heat the oil in a wok over a medium-high heat and fry the beef strips until sealed and browned all over. Add the Chinese five-spice powder, the chilli, onion, garlic and honey and cook for 5 minutes.

2. Add the peanut butter, soy sauce and sesame seeds. Stir well and cook for 2 minutes.

3. Add the mangetout and cooked noodles and mix well. Cook for a further 2 minutes. Stir in the coriander, and serve.

Nutrition: Health score 10.3 High in vitamins B3, B6 and iron

Kcal	Carbs	Sugar	Protein	Fat	Sat Fat	Fibre
715.9	51.6g	9.9g (11.1%)	72.4g	23g	5.7g (28.6%)	5.3g (17.8%)

Sweet Potato Cottage Pie

Serves 1

Prep. 15 minutes

Gluten-free

Feel warmed and cosy even on the coldest of evenings with my well-flavoured, golden cottage pie. It's healthier than the usual recipes because it is vegetable-rich and topped with sweet potato, which lowers the glycaemic index (see page 221) of the dish. This balanced meal is Lean Muscle dominant, but it is suitable for most occasions. If you wish to reduce the calories and saturated fat content, you can swap the beef for turkey, but beef is a good source of iron, creatine and B-vitamins.

115g sweet potato, peeled and cut into chunks

2 carrots, chopped

1 celery stick, chopped

1 beef stock cube

250g lean minced beef

1 onion, chopped

1 garlic clove, crushed, or 1 tsp garlic paste

2 tbsp tomato purée

salt and ground black pepper

1. Preheat the oven to 200°C (180°C fan oven) Gas 6. Cook the sweet potato in a saucepan of boiling water for 10 minutes or until soft. Drain in a colander and return to the pan.

2. Put the carrots and celery in a saucepan and crumble in the beef stock cube. Add enough water to cover, bring to the boil and cook until the veg is tender. Drain in a colander, reserving the stock.

3. Put the beef in a frying pan with the onion and garlic and cook for 5 minutes, stirring to break up any lumps of mince.

4. Add the tomato purée, celery and carrot to the pan, then add half the reserved stock. Bring to the boil, then reduce the heat and simmer for 5 minutes. Season with salt and pepper.

5. Mash the sweet potato and season.

6. Pour the beef mixture into an ovenproof dish and top with the sweet potato mash. Cook in the oven for 25–30 minutes until golden. Serve.

Nutrition: Health Score 7.2 High in Vit B2, Vit A, Vit C & Vit E

Kcal	Carbs	Sugar	Protein	Fat	Sat Fat	Fibre
617.4	46.8g	23.6g (26.2%)	63n	16.?g	6.1y (30%)	14g (36.8%)

Lamb Kefta

Serves 4

Prep. 16 minutes

Gluten-free

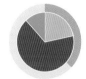

This lamb dish is a real show-stopper. Lamb is a beautifully tender meat, and cooked with a tomato and chilli base ensures that it is mouth-wateringly moist and richly flavoured. Red meat is a good source of haem iron, which is the easiest form of iron for the body to absorb. Lamb is naturally high in fat, so make sure you purchase a better quality of minced lamb to ensure it is lean. The tomato and chilli contain lycopene, which is good for heart health.

500g lean minced lamb

1 tbsp paprika

1 tbsp ground cumin

1 red chilli, seeded and chopped, plus sliced chilli to garnish

juice of ½ lemon

1 red onion, chopped

2 tbsp chopped fresh coriander, plus extra to garnish

400g can plum tomatoes

1 tbsp olive oil

salt and ground black pepper

1. Put the lamb in a bowl and add the remaining ingredients except for the tomatoes and oil. Season with salt and pepper and mix well. Divide into eight and shape into flat rectangles.

2. Heat the oil in a large frying pan over a medium-high heat. Cook the keftas for 2 minutes on each side, turning carefully.

3. Add the tomatoes and bring to the boil, season, then reduce the heat and simmer for 12 minutes or until cooked through. Sprinkle with sliced chilli and coriander, and serve.

Nutrition: Health score 2.3 High in vitamins B1, A and C

Kcal	Carbs	Sugar	Protein	Fat	Sat Fat	Fibre
336.3	5.8g	4.7g (5.2%)	33.1g	19.5g	8.4g (42%)	3.3g (11.1%)

Doner Kebab

Serves 3

Prep. 18 minutes

Could a doner kebab possibly be good for you? Believe me, this one is and it is absolutely delicious. Lamb is a fairly fatty meat, but the boiling method used here means that the calories are reduced but the meat remains lovely and moist. It is a mainly Lean Muscle-based dish but the flatbread provides Fuel and the salad adds Health. It has an impressive health profile with several elements that aid energy metabolism and immunity. Put these out for dinner or a party and you'll be the host with the most.

500g minced lamb

¼ tsp ground black pepper

½ tsp salt

1 tsp smoked paprika

1 tsp ground coriander

1 tsp ground cumin

1 tsp dried oregano

4 garlic cloves, crushed, or 4 tsp garlic paste

¼ tsp ground black pepper

½ tsp salt

1 egg, beaten

3 wholemeal flatbreads, to serve

For the salad:

¼ iceberg lettuce, shredded

1 large tomato, sliced

½ cucumber, sliced

1. Put the lamb in a large bowl and add the remaining ingredients. Mix together well, using your hands if necessary, then form into a large sausage shape and wrap tightly in clingfilm.

2. Bring a large saucepan of water to the boil, then reduce to a simmer. Put the wrapped kebab mixture into the water, cover with the lid and simmer for 30 minutes.

3. Meanwhile, mix the salad ingredients together in a bowl.

4. Remove the kebab from water and unwrap it, then allow it to cool slightly before slicing thinly. Fill the flatbreads with the kebab meat and salad. Serve.

Nutrition: Health score 6.5 High in vitamin B12, iron and zinc

Kcal	Carbs	Sugar	Protein	Fat	Sat Fat	Fibre
366	13.8g	3.8g (4.3%)	45.8g	12.5g	3.5g (17.5%)	9.1g (30.3%)

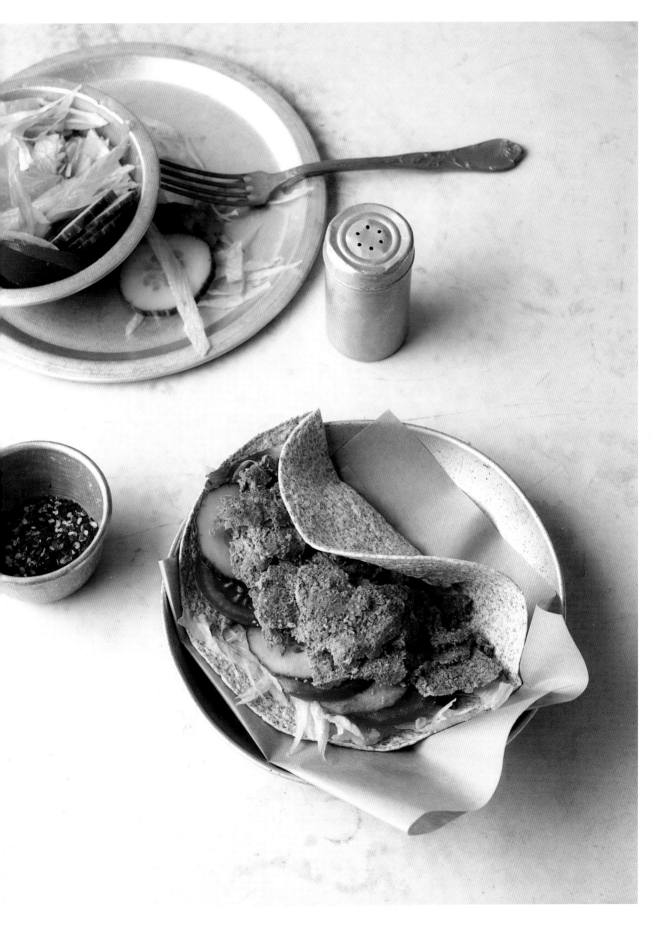

Moussaka

Serves 4

Prep. 18 minutes

Gluten-free

The Mediterranean and Middle Eastern favourite, moussaka, is traditionally made with aubergines and potatoes, but here I have added courgettes and broccoli to upgrade it to a wonderfully healthy and balanced dish. The potatoes and other veg make it a Fuel-dominant meal, but there is lots of protein from the lamb and Greek yogurt, too. The use of yogurt and feta cheese also means that there is less fat and calories than the traditional version, making it suitable for almost any occasion – although it is especially great to aid a rapid recovery.

300g potatoes, peeled

2 aubergines, sliced

olive oil spray

½ onion, chopped

250g low-fat minced beef

250g lean minced lamb

3 garlic cloves, crushed, or 3 tsp garlic paste

2 tbsp dried oregano

400g passata

2 courgettes, sliced

180g low-fat Greek yogurt

1 egg

50g low-fat feta cheese

40g low-fat Cheddar cheese, grated

300g broccoli, cut into florets and steamed, to serve

1. Cook the potatoes in a saucepan of boiling water for 15 minutes or until tender. Drain in a colander, then slice thickly.

2. Preheat the oven to 240°C (220°C fan oven) Gas 9 and line a large baking sheet with baking paper. Put the aubergine slices in a layer on the baking sheet and spray with oil. Cook in the oven for 10 minutes or until softened. Set aside.

3. Heat a saucepan over a medium heat and spray with oil. Add the onion, beef and lamb, garlic and oregano, and cook for 3 minutes, stirring occasionally.

4. Add the potato, passata and courgettes, and cook for 5 minutes.

5. Spoon the sauce into an ovenproof dish and cover with the aubergine slices.

6. Put the yogurt in a small bowl and beat in the egg. Spoon evenly over the aubergine slices. Sprinkle with the cheeses and bake for 15 minutes or until golden. Serve with steamed broccoli.

Nutrition: Health score 5.6 High in vitamins B6, B12 and phosphorus

Kcal	Carbs	Sugar	Protein	Fat	Sat Fat	Fibre
539.6	41.5g	20.4g (22.6%)	38.4g	21.7g	9g (45.1%)	13.1g (43.6%)

Minute Steak with Roasted Peppers and Avocado Salad

Serves 2

Prep. 10 minutes

Gluten-free

My Mexican-inspired salad is the perfect taste and texture contrast to go with grilled steak to make a swift and appetising meal. Because the dish is high in protein, it's ideal for those wanting to reduce their carbs, although it still retains a decent calorie load. The meal contains iron – an important nutrient to develop red blood cells, which carry oxygen within the body for energy – and vitamin C, which increases iron's absorption. Avocados are a nutritional powerhouse with a range of vitamins, minerals and healthy monounsaturated fats.

½ red onion, diced

2 red peppers, seeded and diced

2 tbsp olive oil, plus extra to drizzle and fry

grated zest and juice of 1 lemon

1 avocado

100g canned sweetcorn, drained and rinsed

2 minute steaks

salt and ground black pepper

1. Preheat the oven to 180°C (160°C fan oven) Gas 4. Put the diced onion and peppers in a baking tray. Season with salt and pepper and drizzle over a little olive oil. Roast for 15 minutes.

2. Meanwhile, put the lemon zest and juice in a bowl and add the 2 tbsp olive oil. Whisk well.

3. Cut the avocado in half and remove the pit. Scoop out the flesh using a spoon and cut into dice. Add the avocado, sweetcorn, and roasted pepper and onion to the bowl, then mix well.

4. Heat a little oil in a frying pan over a medium-high heat and fry the steaks for 2 minutes on each side or to your liking. Serve the steak with the salad.

Nutrition: Health score 5.7 High in vitamins A, C and folate

Kcal	Carbs	Sugar	Protein	Fat	Sat Fat	Fibre
632.8	17.3g	10.9g (12.1%)	67.6g	30.1g	4.7g (23.6%)	9.9g (33.1%)

Stir-Fry Meal Builder

If you offered me one type of meal for the rest of my life, it would undoubtedly be stir-fries. Endlessly versatile, they are quick, nutritious and delicious. Getting the kids involved in the cooking is a great way to get them to try vegetables. Here's how to go about building your own favourites, with an at-a-glance guide opposite.

- Prepping your ingredients first can be useful, as stir-fries often cook quickly, but with a bit of practice you can normally prep as you go along. Heat a healthy oil, such as olive oil or rapeseed oil, in a large pan or wok.

- If you are adding onion, chop and cook this first for 5 minutes or until it has softened. If using meat or tofu, chop into chunks and cook, turning regularly, for 5–6 minutes until the meat is cooked through. Many recipes add seasoning at this point to flavour the protein.

- Next, add any number of vegetables and salad veg, such as spring onions and peppers, for health. Vegetables that have a root or thicker skins tend to need slightly longer to cook, but all should be done by 6 minutes if chopped thinly.

- Next, it is typical to add some Fuel elements, such as noodles or rice, or to cook them separately. Pre-cooked versions are very handy to just throw in.

- Add a garnish if you like, of nuts, seeds or herbs.

- Finally, add the all-important sauce. You can purchase a vast array of ready-made sources, but homemade ones, such as the those suggested in the infographic, are simple, tasty and typically healthier. Mix the sauce through the stir-fry and cook for 1–2 minutes before serving.

PERFORMANCE
FUEL

LEAN
MUSCLE

HEALTH

1. Heat oil   2. Add sliced protein with chopped aromatics and/or seasoning

Heat oil (coconut, olive, rapeseed) in a pan on medium / high heat

 Chicken or turkey

 Lean steak

 Squid

 Garlic

 Onion

Ginger

Chilli

 Meaty fish
haddock, monkfish, tuna

 Prawn

 Tofu or tempeh

 Salt and pepper

 Cajun, paprika, 5-spice

 Curry spice, curry powder, turmeric

Stir for 3-5 mins

3. Add sliced vegetable and salad items

Cook for 2-5 mins

 Peppers

 Carrot

 Broccoli

 Pak choi

 Beans

 Corn

Asparagus

Cook for 1-2 mins

 Aubergine

 Courgette

 Spinach/kale

 Mushroom

 Beansprout

 Spring onion

4. Add pre- or quick- cook carbs   5. Optional garnish

 Basmati rice or quinoa

 Wholemeal noodles

Beansprouts or vegetable noodles
e.g. courgetti

 Beans
black, kidney, mung

Seeds
sesame, pumpkin, chia, flax

 Nuts
walnut, almond, pistachio

Herbs
coriander, mint, basil, parsley

6. Add pre-made or homemade sauce

Pre-made
szechuan, sweet and sour, chow main, sweet chilli, Thai

Black bean
3 tbsp light soy sauce, 1 tsp ginger, ½ tsp crushed garlic

Sweet and sour
1 tbsp light soy, 2 tbsp rice vinegar, 1 tsp honey

Thai red
coconut milk, 2 tbsp red curry paste, 2 tbsp fish sauce, 1 tsp crushed garlic

Tray Roast Meal Builder

Tray roasts are a really simple and a healthy way to cook a main meal. The prep work is normally done all together, taking under 10 minutes, and then you can just relax, and leave it to cook. Here are the steps, with a handy at-a-glance guide opposite.

- The starting point is to preheat the oven to 180°C (160°C fan oven) Gas 4.

- If you're using larger whole potatoes or root veg you may need to par-boil these first for about 15 minutes, or chop them into small chunks.

- While the oven is heating, prepare your Lean Muscle from protein, Health from vegetables and Fuel from root vegetables. Vary the amounts to suit your goals.

- Spread a healthy oil, such as olive oil, on the base of a roasting tin to prevent sticking and arrange the ingredients evenly over the base. (Alternatively, some recipes use a foil envelope around the ingredients to increase the moisture and steam the ingredients in the flavours.)

- The key to the dish is the seasoning. This can be as simple as a spice such as Cajun or paprika for a bit of heat, or balsamic vinegar or lemon juice for sharpness. Some simple marinades are shown on the infographic or you can buy a pre-made one. Spread over the ingredients, then pop your tray roast in the oven and relax for 20–25 minutes until it is cooked through and golden. If cooking a large breast of chicken whole, you might need to cook it for slightly longer and remember to check it is cooked through by piercing it with a knife to ensure that the juices run clear.

PERFORMANCE
FUEL

LEAN
MUSCLE

HEALTH

1. Pre-heat oven

180°C
(160°C fan oven)
Gas 4

2. Choose and prepare your protein

Salmon

Chicken or turkey

Lean beef

Meaty fish
sea bass, monkfish

Vegan or vegetarian
sausages

Tofu or tempeh

3. Prepare vegetables

Peppers

Carrot

Broccoli

Cauliflower

Onion

Asparagus

Aubergine

Courgette

Beans

Mushroom

Corn

Tomatoes

4. Prepare the carbs

Sweet
potato

Butternut
squash

New
potatoes

Parsnip

Turnip

5. Prepare baking tray

Add oil to a baking
tray or use foil
parcel to maintain
moisture. Arrange the
ingredients

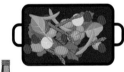

6. Cover with seasoning/flavouring

Sharp soy
2 tbsp balsamic
2 tbsp lemon
2 tbsp soy
sauce
2 tbsp olive oil
1 tsp chilli
flakes

Spicy garlic
2 tbsp garlic
2 tbsp paprika

Italian
2 tbsp garlic
1 tbsp rosmary
2 tbsp thyme

Honey glaze
3 tbsp honey
2 tbsp lemon
1 tbsp olive oil

Sauces
balsamic,
sweet chilli,
soy sauce,
BBQ

Seasoning
salt and
pepper, cajun,
paprika,
5-spice,
oregano,
Italian, garlic

Herbs
thyme, basil,
mint, rosemary

7. Cook

Cook for
25-30 mins

SIDE DISHES

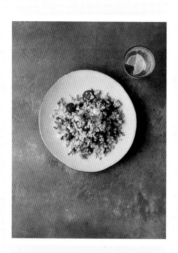

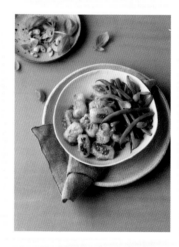

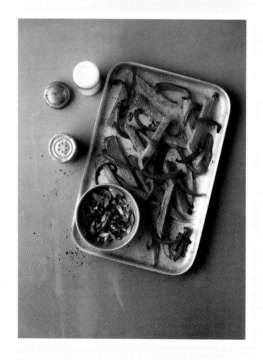

Spiced Bulgur Wheat

Serves 3

Prep. 10 minutes

Vegan

Enjoy this carb side dish for a tasty change from the ordinary – it packs more flavour and health than your run-of-the-mill carb accompaniment. Bulgur wheat has more fibre and protein but fewer calories than standard carb side dishes, such as potatoes and pasta. This dish also packs a host of micronutrients including vitamins A and C from the carrot and pepper. The stock and curry powder provide bags of flavour, so you won't crave an additional sauce.

200ml vegetable stock

100g bulgur wheat

1 tbsp olive oil

1 tsp curry powder

1 carrot, finely chopped

1 green pepper, seeded and finely chopped

½ red onion, finely chopped

100g canned sweetcorn, drained and rinsed

4 tbsp fresh chopped coriander

salt and ground black pepper

1. Put the stock in a large saucepan and bring to the boil, then reduce the heat to a simmer. Add the bulgur wheat and bring back to a simmer, then cook for 10 minutes.

2. Add the olive oil, curry powder and vegetables. Season with salt and pepper. Cook for 5 minutes or until tender. Add the coriander, mix well and serve.

Nutrition: Health score 3.6 High in vitamins A and C

Kcal	Carbs	Sugar	Protein	Fat	Sat Fat	Fibre
136.3	14.7g	6.4g (7.1%)	2.9g	5.8g	0.9g (4.7%)	4.6g (12.2%)

Cabbage Salad

Serves 2

Prep. 8 minutes

Vegan, gluten-free

When I tried this dish I could not believe how much I enjoyed it. It is so simple and quick – and weirdly moreish. Cabbage is full of vitamin K and anthocyanins, which help with mental function and concentration, in addition to vitamins A and C. Chillies are anti-inflammatory and, along with the lemon, give the salad that kick that draws you back for more. It is a low-calorie, high-fibre side dish, great for those trying to lose weight.

½ white cabbage

1 onion

½–1 red chilli, to taste, seeded

a few sprigs of parsley and basil, leaves chopped

juice of 1–2 lemons, to taste

olive oil

salt and ground black pepper

1. Put the cabbage, onion and chilli in a food processor and shred finely. (Alternatively, shred using a sharp knife.)

2. Tip into a bowl. Add the parsley, basil and lemon juice. Drizzle with the oil and season with salt and pepper.

3. Scrunch the mixture together using your hands, then serve.

Nutrition: Health score 8.1 High in vitamins A, C, K and protein

Kcal	Carbs	Sugar	Protein	Fat	Sat Fat	Fibre
151.7	21.3g	16g (17.7%)	6g	2.9g	0.5g (2.4%)	10.3g (27%)

Curried Cauli Rice

Serves 2

Prep. 8 minutes

Vegan and gluten-free

Cauli rice has become a popular low-carb side choice for those looking to lose weight. It looks and functions like rice, soaking up the flavours of the accompanying dish but without the calories and carbs. Cauliflower is a good source of vitamin C, and turmeric has been found to have powerful anti-inflammatory properties, in addition to giving the 'rice' a nice spicy flavour. You can buy pre-packaged quick-cook cauli rice, but as this version is so easy to make, why bother?

½ cauliflower

1 tbsp olive oil

1 tsp curry powder

1 tsp ground turmeric

salt and ground black pepper

1. Cut the cauliflower into rough chunks and put into a food processor. Blitz until finely chopped like grains of rice. (Alternatively, put the cauliflower on a large chopping board and, using a large, sharp knife, slice down through the florets to chop the cauliflower finely.)

2. Heat the oil in a frying pan over a medium heat, then add the cauli rice. Cook for 4 minutes, stirring regularly, until soft. Season with salt and pepper.

3. Stir in the curry powder and turmeric, and cook for a further 2 minutes. Serve.

Nutrition: Health score 2.8 High in vitamin C and curcumin

Kcal	Carbs	Sugar	Protein	Fat	Sat Fat	Fibre
92	1.8g	1.1g (1.3%)	2.5g	7.2g	1g (5.1%)	4.5g (11.9%)

Tabbouleh

Serves 2

Prep. 5 minutes

Vegan

Originating in the Levant in the Middle East, tabbouleh is a refreshing vegan salad made with bulgur wheat, herbs and vegetables. The bulgur wheat is a relatively low glycaemic index carb (see page 221) with a good complement of fibre and B vitamins. The spring onions and cherry tomatoes add some Health, but it is the herbs that steal the show, making this Fuel-based salad a firm favourite.

100g bulgur wheat

grated zest and juice of ½ lemon

¼ cucumber, finely diced

2 spring onions, finely chopped

1 tsp chopped fresh coriander

1 tsp chopped fresh parsley

1 tsp chopped fresh mint

2 tbsp olive oil

6 cherry tomatoes, quartered

salt and ground black pepper

1. Cook the bulgur wheat in a saucepan with twice the quantity of boiling water for 12 minutes, then cover and leave for 10 minutes, or according to the pack instructions. Drain in a sieve and transfer to a bowl.

2. Use a fork to fluff up the bulgur wheat, then add the remaining ingredients. Season with salt and pepper. Combine well, then serve.

Nutrition: Health score 2.7 High in vitamins A and K

Kcal	Carbs	Sugar	Protein	Fat	Sat Fat	Fibre
224.7	18.5g	2.8g (3.1%)	2.8g	15.3g	2.1g (10.5%)	2.9g (9.6%)

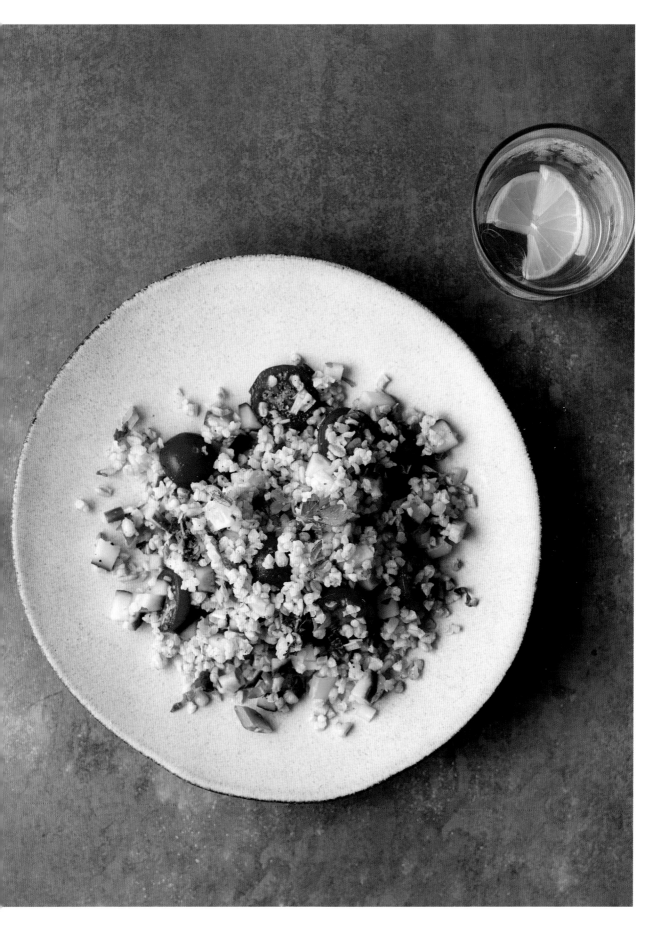

Cajun Street Rice

Serves 2

Prep. 20 minutes

Gluten-free

Capture the flavours of mouthwatering Asian street food with this simple dish. It's a wonderfully balanced meal with carbs and protein, and it also possesses lots of health benefits, so it's great for almost all occasions but especially good to promote recovery. We have used minced turkey to reduce the saturated fat content, and the carrot, onions and peppers provide high amounts of vitamins A, C and K, in addition to adding to the lovely textures and flavours. It's a favourite in our house as a side dish or main meal. The quantities given serve 2 as a main but 4 as a side dish.

200g brown basmati rice

1 beef stock cube

1 bay leaf

olive oil spray

400g minced turkey

½ onion, finely chopped

4 rashers back bacon, chopped

2 tsp Cajun seasoning

1 tsp Worcestershire sauce

1 carrot, finely chopped

6 mushrooms, sliced

½ red pepper, seeded and chopped

½ green pepper, seeded and chopped

a small bunch of spring onions, finely sliced

1. To cook the rice, boil a large pan of water. Rinse the rice thoroughly in a sieve and add it to the water. Boil for 20–25 minutes or until tender, or according to the pack instructions. Drain in a colander.

2. Crumble the stock cube into a jug and add the bay leaf and 200ml (scant 1 cup) boiling water. Set aside.

3. Spray a saucepan with oil spray and heat over a medium heat. Add the turkey, onion and bacon, and cook for 3–4 minutes, stirring, until brown.

4. Add the Cajun seasoning and Worcestershire sauce, and stir, then add the carrot, mushrooms and peppers. Pour in the beef stock, then cook for 4 minutes.

5. Add the cooked rice and spring onions to the pan and stir over a medium heat until the rice is coated. Serve.

Nutrition: Health score 6.9 High in vitamins A, B6 and C

Kcal	Carbs	Sugar	Protein	Fat	Sat Fat	Fibre
504.5	40.2g	8.6g (9.6%)	47.4g	15.6g	5.1g (25.7%)	4.6g (15.2%)

Loaded But Light Potato Skins

Serves 4

Prep. 15 minutes

Gluten-free

Many people love to eat loaded potato skins, so we've adapted the recipe to keep the great taste but made them far healthier, reducing the saturated fat content and calories. They are predominantly a Fuel choice due to the potatoes, but they contain a decent amount of protein from the cottage cheese, and Health is boosted with a range of vitamins, minerals and fibre. The calories are only moderate, so they are suitable for most occasions as a side or a full meal if you fancy a few.

4 baking potatoes, skins scrubbed, dried

5 spring onions, finely chopped

2 ham slices, chopped

200g low-fat cottage cheese

30g Parmesan, grated

salt and ground black pepper

1. Pierce the potatoes all over with a fork. Microwave for 4 minutes, then use tongs to turn them and cook for a further 3 minutes or until soft when squeezed when held in a tea towel.

2. Preheat the oven to 220°C (200°C fan oven) Gas 7. Cut each potato in half and scoop out the potato into a bowl.

3. Mash the potato using a fork, then stir in the spring onions, ham and cottage cheese. Season with salt and pepper.

4. Spoon the mixture back into the skins, and sprinkle with Parmesan. Put on a baking sheet and cook for 20 minutes until the topping is golden.

Nutrition: Health score 4.1 High in vitamin B6, copper and iron

Kcal	Carbs	Sugar	Protein	Fat	Sat Fat	Fibre
266	34.6g	4.2g (4.7%)	15.3g	5.6g	2.5g (12.3%)	5.1g (16.9%)

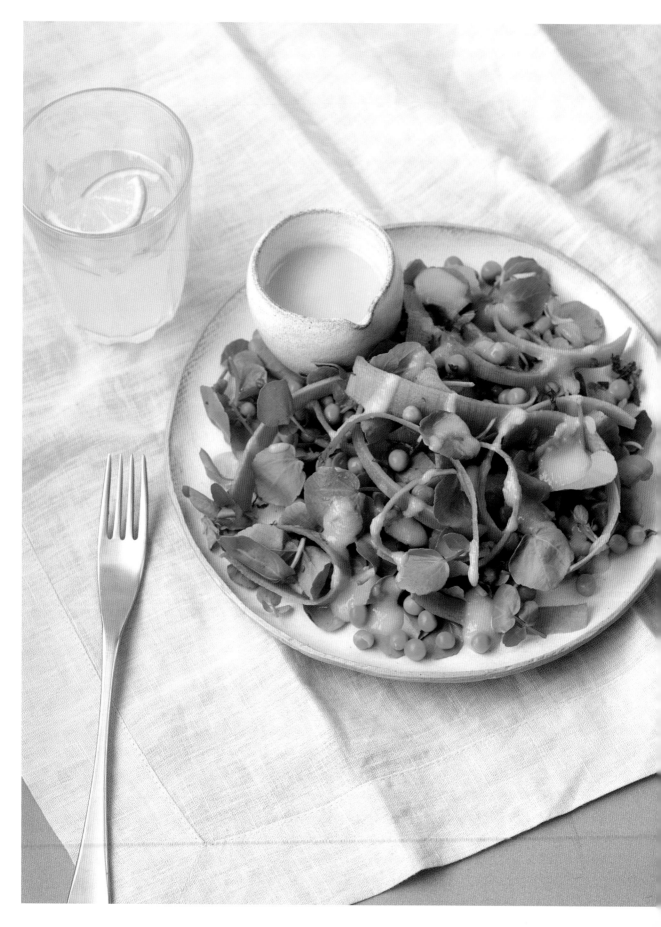

Pea, Watercress and Carrot Salad

Serves 4

Prep. 8 minutes

Vegan, gluten-free

This original salad is freshness itself with a beautiful fruity dressing. Not only super-easy to make but it also offers numerous health benefits. The carrots provide over 100 per cent of the RDA of vitamin A, which is important for the eyesight, and the peas, watercress and mango provide vitamins C and E, excellent for immunity and skin health. The mango dressing is delicious and leaves you craving more, but as it's low in calories and high in fibre it makes a great choice for weight management.

150g frozen peas

1 mango

50ml olive oil

2 tbsp white wine vinegar

2 carrots

100g watercress

2 sprigs of fresh mint, leaves chopped

1. Put the peas in a saucepan and add boiling water to cover. Bring to the boil and cook for 5 minutes. Drain in a colander, then rinse under cold water and drain again. Set aside.

2. Using a sharp knife, cut each side of the mango away from the large pit in the centre. Score rough squares into the mango flesh and then push the skin side inwards to make the mango cubes stand proud. Cut off the cubes. Cut off the flesh around the pit. Put the mango into a food processor or blender and add the olive oil and vinegar, then blitz until smooth.

3. Use a vegetable peeler to cut the carrots into strips.

4. Put the peas, carrots, watercress and mint in a bowl. Add the mango dressing and season with salt and pepper to taste. Serve.

Nutrition: Health score 6.8 High in vitamins A, B3 and B12

Kcal	Carbs	Sugar	Protein	Fat	Sat Fat	Fibre
242.9	17.5g	14.9g (16.5%)	3.5g	16.7g	1.9g (11.8%)	3.7g (12.4%)

Balsamic Kale

Serves 1
—
Prep. 3 minutes
—
Vegan, gluten-free
—

Kale is one of the most nutrient-dense foods around: it is high in vitamins A, C and K, and contains the flavonoids quercetin and kaempferol. These nutrients have numerous health benefits for your heart, inflammation and immunity. Kale is also high in fibre and therefore great for gut health. The only issue is that it can be a bit bland – but not in this recipe, which adds loads of flavour. It's super-quick and simple to make and a great side dish or addition to a salad.

1 tbsp olive oil

2 tbsp balsamic vinegar

1 tsp brown sugar

100g kale, shredded

salt and ground black pepper

1. Put the oil in a saucepan over a medium heat and add the vinegar and sugar. Stir until the sugar dissolves.

2. Add the kale and stir through the sauce. Cook for 4 minutes, then season and serve.

Nutrition: Health score 12.6 High in vitamins A, C and K

Kcal	Carbs	Sugar	Protein	Fat	Sat Fat	Fibre
213.8	15.1g	11.5g (12.7%)	4.4g	14.4g	2g (9.8%)	3.6g (12%)

Leeks, Peas and Quinoa

Serves 2

Prep. 12 minutes

Vegan, gluten-free

This super-grain side dish provides a carbohydrate-rich boost to any main meal. Quinoa provides a complete protein source, as it contains all the essential amino acids to support muscle repair and remodelling, and it is packed with fibre to help control energy levels and maintain a healthy digestive system. Leeks, like all the members of the onion family, contain allicin, which helps to reduce inflammation, and peas are a great source of vitamin C.

2 tbsp olive oil, plus extra for drizzling

1–2 leeks, chopped

1 bag of microwave quinoa

125g frozen peas

1 vegetable or chicken stock cube

salt and ground black pepper

1. Heat the oil in a saucepan over a medium heat and cook the leeks for 2 minutes.

2. Meanwhile, microwave the quinoa according to the pack instructions.

3. Put the peas in a saucepan and add boiling water to cover. Bring to the boil and cook for 4 minutes. Drain in a colander.

4. Add the quinoa and peas to the pan with the leeks. Crumble over the stock cube and splash over some more oil and 2 tablespoons of water. Season with salt and pepper. Cook for 1–2 minutes, stirring occasionally.

Nutrition: Health score 7.5 High in vitamins B1, A, K and manganese

Kcal	Carbs	Sugar	Protein	Fat	Sat Fat	Fibre
382	57.5g	9.8g (10.9%)	16g	5.9g	0.6g (2.9%)	9.7g (25.4%)

Salt and Pepper Sweet Potato Chips

Serves 2

Prep. 5 minutes

Vegan, gluten-free

Put down the takeaway menus and step into the kitchen to make these delicious sweet potato chips. They are full of flavour, although they contain minimal fat and their other health benefits include good quantities of iron and vitamin C, which act in combination to help to support our immune system and fight off infections.

olive oil spray

2 large sweet potatoes, peeled and cut into chips

½ red pepper, seeded and cut into thin strips

½ green pepper, seeded and cut into thin strips

3 spring onions, thinly sliced

1 medium chilli, thinly sliced

½ tsp chilli flakes

½ tsp Chinese five-spice powder

1 garlic clove, crushed, or 1 tsp garlic paste

salt and ground black pepper

1. Preheat the oven to 220°C (200°C fan oven) Gas 7. Spray a baking tray with olive oil, then put the sweet potato chips on the tray.

2. Add the peppers, season with salt and pepper and spray with a little more oil. Roast for 20 minutes.

3. Meanwhile, put the spring onions in a bowl and add the chilli, five-spice powder and garlic. Mix well. Once the sweet potato is cooked, add it to the bowl and toss well to mix. Serve.

Nutrition: Health score 4.5 High in vitamins B5, C, K and manganese

Kcal	Carbs	Sugar	Protein	Fat	Sat Fat	Fibre
197	36.4g	15.6g (17.4%)	5g	0.8g	0.2g (0.9%)	8.2g (21.7%)

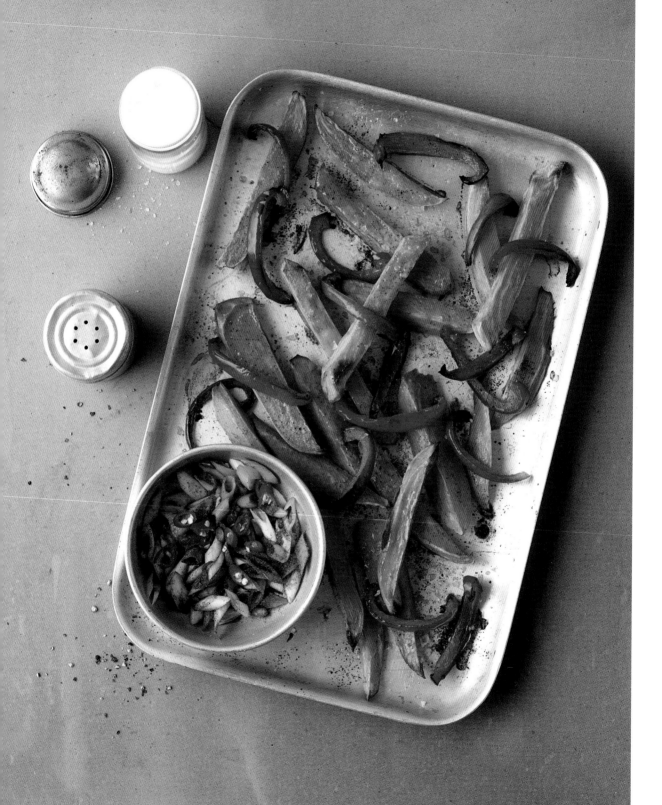

Mushroom Bruschetta

Serves 1

Prep. 10 minutes

Vegan

The classic Italian starter, bruschetta, is always popular because it looks so appetising – and tastes great with the garlic-infused bread and topping of mushrooms. The bread makes this a predominant Fuel meal, but the mushrooms provide copper and selenium, which are good for our immune system. Easy to make, this is fantastic as a side dish or snack.

1 tsp olive oil

40g button mushrooms, sliced

1 small ciabatta, cut in half

2 garlic cloves, crushed, or 2 tsp garlic paste

1. Preheat the grill. Heat the oil in a frying pan and cook the mushrooms for 5 minutes, turning regularly.

2. Spread the garlic paste over each half of ciabatta and scatter over the mushrooms. Grill for 2 minutes or until golden. Serve.

Nutrition: Health score 2.4 High in folate, copper and selenium

Kcal	Carbs	Sugar	Protein	Fat	Sat Fat	Fibre
231.3	33.5g	4.8g (5.4%)	7g	6.7g	0.7g (3.4%)	3.1g (10.2%)

Roasted Vegetables

Serves 2

Prep. 10 minutes

Vegan, gluten-free

Colourful and appetising, this selection of vegetables roasted with olive oil and whole garlic cloves smells as good as it looks. What better way to eat your five-a-day, which provide a whole host of nutrients and phytochemicals to keep you fit and healthy? To seal the deal, the dish couldn't be easier to put together.

your choice of vegetables, such as peppers, shallots, green beans, tomatoes, broccoli, cauliflower, asparagus and carrots, chopped into chunky pieces

6 garlic cloves, peeled but left whole

1 tsp dried oregano

a drizzle of olive oil

drizzle of balsamic vinegar (optional)

roast vegetable seasoning, or salt and ground black pepper

1. Preheat the oven to 200°C (180°C fan oven) Gas 6. Put all the veg in large roasting tin and add the garlic and oregano. Drizzle with the olive oil and balsamic, if using.

2. Add the seasoning and mix with the vegetables. Spread them evenly in the tin. Roast for 20–25 minutes until golden. Serve.

Nutrition: Health score 5.2 High in vitamins B6, C, fibre and manganese

Kcal	Carbs	Sugar	Protein	Fat	Sat Fat	Fibre
229.5	30g	17.2g (19.1%)	4.9g	7.9g	1.2g (5.8%)	11.1g (29.2%)

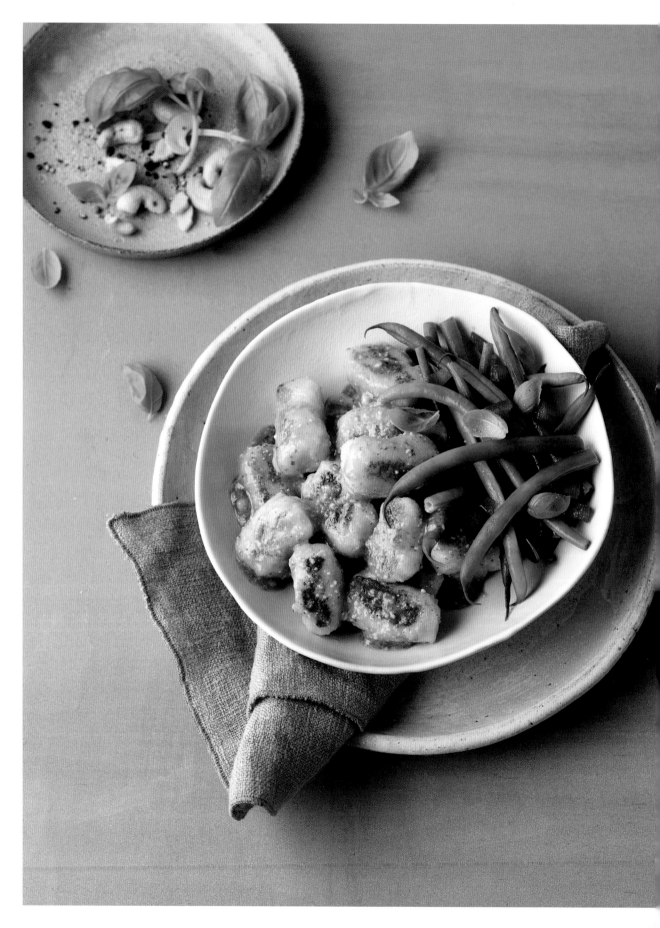

Basil Pesto Gnocchi

Serves 2

Prep. 10 minutes

Vegan

Gnocchi is an Italian favourite, so we've created a version that is super-easy to make, healthy and, above all, it tastes perfect! It is high in carbs but also protein and a number of minerals. The basil pesto provides bags of flavour and healthy fats. Eat as a side or main dish. If eating as a main, try it with green beans and chopped tomatoes – *bellissimo!*

300g potatoes, cut into chunks

60g pasta flour

2 tbsp basil leaves

50g cashew nuts

1 garlic clove, crushed, or 1 tsp garlic paste

2 tbsp olive oil

1. Cook the potatoes in a saucepan of boiling water for 15 minutes or until tender. Drain in a colander, then briefly return them to the pan over a very low heat to dry off any remaining moisture.

2. Mash the potatoes until smooth, then sieve in the flour. Mix together well.

3. Use your hands to form a ball of the dough, then roll it into a sausage shape. Cut the rolled dough into small squares.

4. Put the basil into a food processor or blender and add the nuts, garlic and 1 tbsp of the oil. Blitz until smooth. Set aside.

5. Bring a large saucepan of water to the boil, then add the gnocchi squares. Cook until they rise to the surface and float. Remove from the pan using a slotted spoon.

6. Heat the remaining 1 tbsp oil in a frying pan over a medium-high heat and fry the gnocchi until brown on both sides. Put into a bowl.

7. Pour the pesto over the gnocchi and gently mix until combined. Serve.

Nutrition: Health score 4.2 High in vitamin B6, copper and iron

Kcal	Carbs	Sugar	Protein	Fat	Sat Fat	Fibre
412.1	31.5g	3g (3.3%)	20.9g	19.7g	2.9g (14.6%)	9.8g (32.6%)

Ratatouille

Serves 2

Prep. 10 minutes

Vegan, gluten-free

Enjoy this super-healthy Italian vegan dish, which is not only rich and tasty but also counts as three of your five-a-day. The tomato sauce is a dietary source of the antioxidant lycopene, which possesses an array of health benefits, including a reduction in the risk of heart disease and cancer. The onion, courgette and garlic are all anti-inflammatory too.

1 tbsp olive oil

½ onion, chopped

1 garlic clove, crushed or 1 tsp garlic paste

1 courgette, cut into small chunks

1 red pepper, seeded and cut into small chunks

400g can chopped tomatoes

1 tbsp dried mixed herbs

salt and ground black pepper

1. Heat the oil in saucepan over a medium heat and cook the onion and garlic for 3 minutes.

2. Add the courgette and pepper to the pan and cook for 5 minutes.

3. Add the tomatoes and herbs, and season with salt and pepper. Bring to the boil, then reduce the heat and simmer for 20 minutes or until the vegetables are soft. Serve.

Nutrition: Health score 4.2 High in vitamins A and C

Kcal	Carbs	Sugar	Protein	Fat	Sat Fat	Fibre
112.7	17.5g	13.5g (15%)	5.2g	0.6g	0.1g (0.5%)	4.7g (15.6%)

Sweet-and-Sour Crispy Asian Sprouts

Serves 4

Prep. 5 minutes

Vegan, gluten-free

Brussels sprouts are a bit like Marmite: you either love them or hate them. This recipe, however, will make you love them because the strong flavours will set your taste buds on fire. Sprouts can be considered a super-food: they are high in antioxidants to help protect against disease; iron and folate to help deliver oxygen to our organs; and fibre to aid gut health.

1kg Brussels sprouts

olive oil spray

4 tsp honey

50ml balsamic vinegar

½ tbsp tamari or dark soy sauce

1 tsp garlic granules

½ vegetable stock cube

1 tsp Chinese five-spice powder

1 tsp chilli powder

1. Preheat the oven to 240°C (220°C fan oven) Gas 9. Put the sprouts on a baking tray and spray them with a couple of squirts of oil. Cook in the oven for 20 minutes.

2. Meanwhile, put the honey in a small saucepan over a high heat and add the vinegar, soy sauce, garlic granules, stock cube, five-spice powder and chilli. Stir until combined then cook until the mixture becomes syrupy.

3. Take the sprouts out of the oven, then pour the syrup over them and toss until the sprouts are evenly covered with the sauce. Serve.

Nutrition: Health score 10 High in vitamins A, B6, C and K

Kcal	Carbs	Sugar	Protein	Fat	Sat Fat	Fibre
146.7	21.6g	13.3g	9.1g	0.9g	0.2g	9.6g
		(14.8%)			(0.9%)	(32.1%)

SNACKS AND DESSERTS

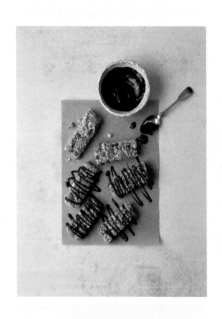

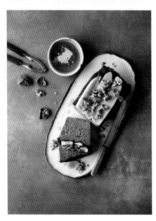

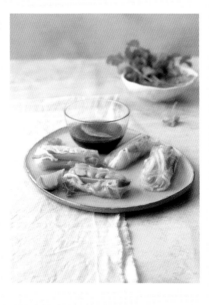

Sushi Rolls

Serves 2

Prep. 8 minutes

These salmon sushi rolls provide bite-sized, all-in-one recovery in an instant! The combination of all three macronutrients is an easy choice for promoting muscle recovery and replenishing depleted energy stores after a hard training session. Plus, the omega-3-rich salmon can help to reduce inflammation and further aid recovery. Dip them in wasabi for an extra kick! (Make sure that you freeze the salmon before using it, to kill any bacteria or parasites.)

1 very fresh salmon fillet, frozen for 24 hours, then thawed

4 tbsp rice vinegar

2 tbsp sesame oil

juice of 1 lime

1 tbsp sriracha

1 tbsp chopped chives

2 nori sheets

100g (1 cup) ready-cooked sushi rice

½ cucumber, sliced

wasabi, to serve (optional)

1. Cut the salmon into small cubes and put into a bowl. Add the rice vinegar, sesame oil, lime juice, sriracha and chopped chives, then mix together well.

2. Take a nori sheet and put it on a sheet of baking paper or use a cane sushi roller to help you roll it. Spread half the sushi rice evenly over the nori, then put half the cucumber slices and salmon on top. Roll up the nori lengthways to form a cylinder. Cut into 4 pieces. Repeat with the second nori sheet. Serve with wasabi, if you like.

Nutrition: Health score 11.8 High in vitamins B2, B3, B5, B6 and B12

Kcal	Carbs	Sugar	Protein	Fat	Sat Fat	Fibre
500	42.2g	2.1g (2.4%)	43.3g	15.4g	2.3g (11.8%)	3.8g (19%)

Lettuce and Tuna Boats

Serves 2

Prep. 8 minutes

Gluten-free

All aboard these punchy tuna boats for a low-carbohydrate snack packed with goodness: vitamin C from the vegetables to support the immune system; and heart-healthy monounsaturated fatty acids from the avocado. Not only this, but we have all your protein needs covered with the fiery tuna filling.

110g can tuna steak, drained

1 tomato, chopped into cubes

1 yellow pepper, seeded and chopped into cubes

1 avocado, halved, pitted and chopped into small cubes

½ red onion, finely chopped

1 red chilli, seeded and chopped

2 tbsp extra virgin olive oil

1 tsp tamari or light soy sauce

8–10 Little Gem lettuce leaves

ground black pepper

1. Put the tuna in a large bowl and add the tomato, yellow pepper, avocado, onion and chilli.

2. Add a little pepper, the oil and soy sauce.

3. Spoon the mixture onto the lettuce leaves. If the lettuce leaves are big, you can fold them to make a wrap around the filling, otherwise leave them open. Serve.

Nutrition: Health score 8.1 High in vitamins B3, B6, B12 and C

Kcal	Carbs	Sugar	Protein	Fat	Sat Fat	Fibre
365.6	11.2g	8.2g (9.1%)	20.7g	24.9g	3.5g (17.6%)	7.4g (24.6%)

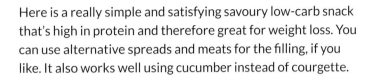

Courgette and Turkey Rolls

Serves 6

Prep. 5 minutes

Here is a really simple and satisfying savoury low-carb snack that's high in protein and therefore great for weight loss. You can use alternative spreads and meats for the filling, if you like. It also works well using cucumber instead of courgette.

1 courgette or cucumber

3 slices (approx. 60g) turkey or chicken slices

4 tbsp low-fat hummus or cheese spread

1. Using a mandolin or knife, cut the courgette into long, thin slices.
2. Slice the meat lengthways into thirds or similar widths to the courgette slices. Lightly spread the hummus on top of the courgette slices, then lay the meat on top.
3. Roll up and secure with a cocktail stick, if you like. Serve.

Nutrition: Health score 0.4 High in copper and manganese

Kcal	Carbs	Sugar	Protein	Fat	Sat Fat	Fibre
79.5	3g	0.9 (1%)	3.2g	6g	0.1g (0.7%)	1.6g (2.4%)

Almond Cobbler

Serves 1

Prep. 3 minutes

Vegetarian, gluten-free

Try this variation on a traditional fruit cobbler, made in a mug in the microwave for the fastest dessert or snack possible. It tastes incredible and provides a good hit of protein, some carbs and a good proportion of Health, including vitamins and healthy fats.

½ banana

20g ground almonds

1 egg

40g (2 scoops) vanilla protein powder

2 tbsp milk

1. Mash the banana and put it into a large mug or ramekin.
2. Put the almonds and the remaining ingredients into the mug. Stir to combine well.
3. Microwave at full power for 2 minutes. Serve, but beware: the cobbler will be *hot*.

Nutrition: Health score 3.0 High in vitamins B2, E and manganese

Kcal	Carbs	Sugar	Protein	Fat	Sat Fat	Fibre
305.7	17.5g	11.9g (13.2%)	22.7g	15.4g	2.7g (13.7%)	3.9g (10.3%)

Edamame Summer Rolls

Serves 2

Prep. 10 minutes

Vegan

Fresh, crunchy and super-easy to make, these Asian-inspired rolls with a dip make a tasty side dish or snack – and they're vegan friendly! They are a good Fuel source and provide many health benefits, including folate, vitamins A and C, and fibre. They're great for parties too!

80g edamame beans

1 small rice noodles nest

8 sheets rice paper

½ red pepper, seeded and cut into thin batons

2 spring onions, cut into thin batons

½ carrot, cut into thin batons

a handful of beansprouts

2 tsp soy sauce

½ tsp garlic granules

1 tsp sesame oil

juice of ½ orange

1. Cook the edamame beans in a small saucepan of boiling water for 2–3 minutes or until tender. Drain in a colander, then refresh under cold water. Set aside.

2. Cook the noodles in a saucepan of boiling water for 4 minutes, or according to the pack instructions. Drain in a colander.

3. Soak a sheet of rice paper in a shallow bowl of hot water for 5 seconds, then lay it on a chopping board.

4. Leaving space around the edges, fill the rice paper with an eighth of the vegetables and a heaped teaspoon of the noodles.

5. Fold up the sides of the rice paper, then fold up the side closest to you and tightly roll it up so that the filling is secure inside and all the edges are sealed. Repeat with the other rice paper sheets.

6. Put the soy sauce in a small bowl and add the garlic granules, oil and orange juice, then whisk well to combine. Serve as a dip with the rolls.

Nutrition: Health score 4.8 High in vitamins A, C and folate

Kcal	Carbs	Sugar	Protein	Fat	Sat Fat	Fibre
261.1	38.6g	8.4g (9.3%)	8.2g	6.1g	0.7g (3.6%)	6.1g (20.5%)

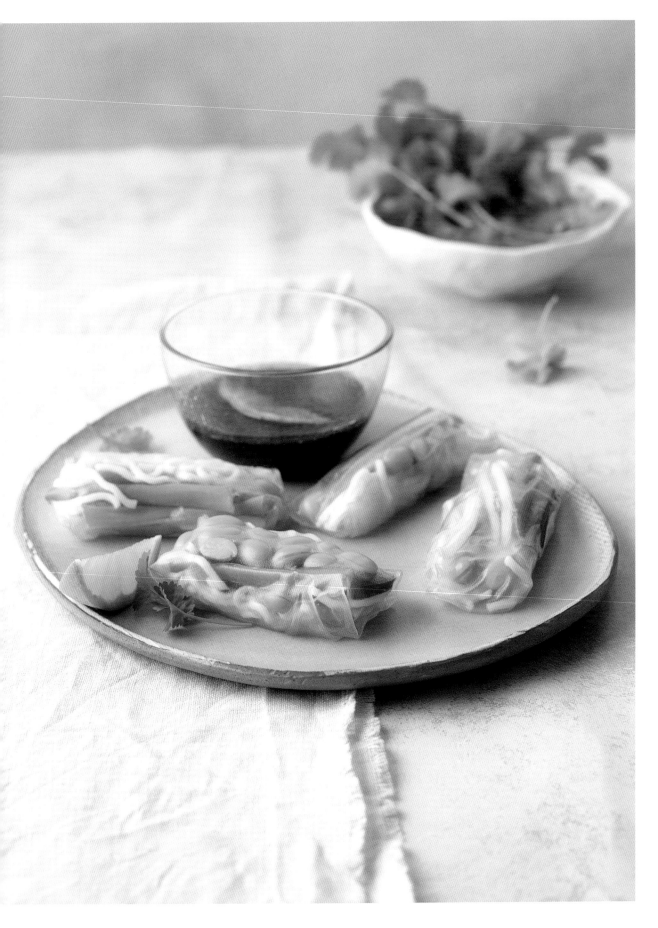

Joint Jellies

Serves 8

Prep. 8 minutes

Gluten-free

Eat these little jellies as a snack or as part of your breakfast. Gelatine is a natural animal product that forms collagen when eaten and helps to support joint and skin health. The vitamin C from the cordial helps with the collagen absorption. These jellies are extremely low in calories but they have a high volume for the amount of calories, which increases satiety, making them great for weight loss.

4 gelatine leaves

560ml diluted cordial of your choice

1. Put the gelatine leaves in bowl of cold water to cover and leave to soak for 5 minutes.
2. Put the diluted cordial in a saucepan and heat gently.
3. Once the gelatine has softened, remove it from the water and squeeze out the excess.
4. Put the gelatine in the cordial mixture and stir until dissolved.
5. Leave to cool, then pour it into eight small pots and chill in the fridge for 45 minutes or until set. Serve.

Nutrition: Health score 11.8 High in collagen

Kcal	Carbs	Sugar	Protein	Fat	Sat Fat	Fibre
18.4	1.5g	1.5g (1.7%)	3g	0.1g	0g (0%)	0g (0%)

Boiled Egg with Hummus and Cucumber

Serves 1

Prep. 8 minutes

Vegetarian

Inspired by Middle Eastern cuisine, this snack provides a great balance of macros and plenty of Health. Arabic flatbread is like a cross between a pitta and a naan, and can be found in many supermarkets. The hummus and eggs contain healthy unsaturated fats, and the chickpeas are a high-fibre fuel source with the added benefit of B vitamins for energy metabolism. Cucumbers are low in calories and high in vitamin K. Although the calorie hit is high for a snack, the high protein and fibre will leave you feeling full for a long time.

3 eggs

1 Arabic flatbread

2 tbsp hummus

¼ large cucumber, cut into batons

1. Put the eggs in a saucepan of boiling water. Return to the boil and cook for 10 minutes. Drain the pan and refill with cold water. Drain and fill again. Leave the eggs to cool, then peel and cut into quarters.

2. Serve the eggs with Arabic bread, hummus and cucumber.

Nutrition: Health score 3.5 High in vitamin B2, B5, B12 and selenium

Kcal	Carbs	Sugar	Protein	Fat	Sat Fat	Fibre
415.8	33.8g	9.6g (10.7%)	21.5g	20.2g	6.5g (32.4%)	3.8g (12.7%)

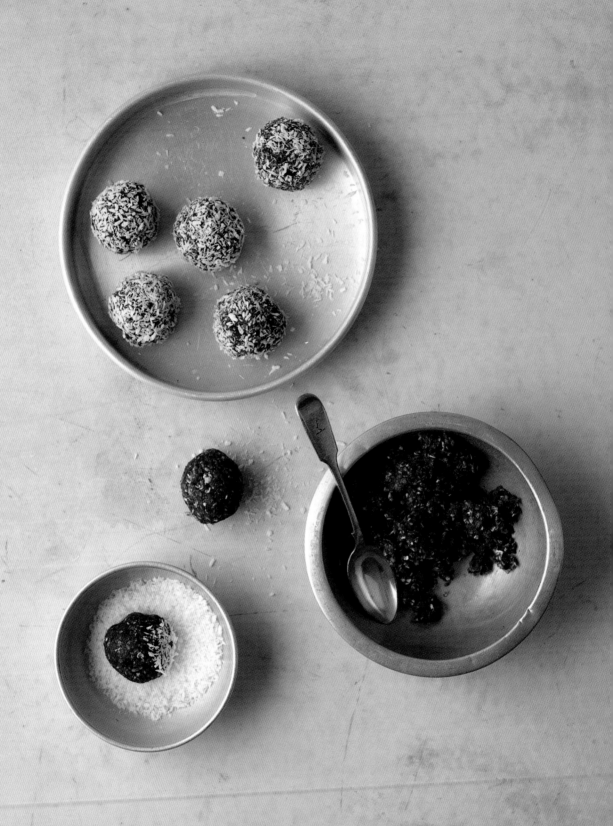

Almond and Berry Balls

Makes 9 servings

Prep. 5 minutes

Vegan, gluten-free

I posted the video for this recipe during the pandemic and it got an incredible reaction as these fruit and nut balls look and taste great. They provide a good hit of carbs, in addition to vitamins B2 and E and magnesium, important for muscle and heart function.

90g pitted dried dates, roughly chopped

125g frozen mixed berries

90g whole blanched almonds

100g (1 cup) porridge oats

10g desiccated coconut

1. Soak the dates in boiling water for 1 minute and drain. Put the berries in a food processor or blender and add the dates. Pulse until the ingredients start to stick together. Scoop out into a bowl. Wipe the blender.

2. Put the almonds in the food processor or blender and blitz to make a fine powder, then add the oats and blitz again until fine.

3. Transfer to the bowl with the berry mixture and mix well. Shape into 9 balls.

4. Put the coconut into a bowl and drop in a ball. Roll it around to coat in the coconut. Repeat with the other balls. Serve.

Nutrition: Health score 1.1 High in vitamins B2, E and magnesium

Kcal	Carbs	Sugar	Protein	Fat	Sat Fat	Fibre
141.5	16g	8.2g (9.1%)	3.7g	6.5g	1.1g (5.7%)	3.5g (11.6%)

Carrot Cake Balls

Makes 8 servings

Prep. 8 minutes

Vegan, gluten-free

I was delighted when we came up with this recipe for energy balls based on the ever-popular carrot cake, as it's my favourite. The oat and date base means that the balls provide a lot of energy, making them great to eat around exercise, plus they transport well, so you can pop them in your gym bag. The carrot provides vitamin A – great for eye and immune health. Dates and coconut also contain several vitamins and minerals.

130g cashew nuts

75g pecan nuts

70g (¾ cup) porridge oats

85g pitted dried dates

115g apple sauce from a jar

1 tbsp (1 scoop) vanilla protein powder, or vegan alternative

1 tbsp ground cinnamon

1 tsp freshly grated nutmeg

1 carrot, grated

30g desiccated coconut

1. Put the cashew nuts in a food processor or blender, and add the pecan nuts, oats, dates, apple sauce, protein powder and spices. Blitz until a dough forms.

2. Add the carrot and blend into the mix, then transfer to a bowl. Put in the fridge for 20–30 minutes to set.

3. Roll the dough into 8 balls. Put the coconut into a bowl and drop in a ball. Roll it around to coat in the coconut. Repeat with the other balls. Serve.

Nutrition: Health score 2.7 High in vitamin A, copper and manganese

Kcal	Carbs	Sugar	Protein	Fat	Sat Fat	Fibre
260.6	21.3g	12g (13.3%)	8.1g	16g	3.2g (15.9%)	3.7g (9.6%)

Mango and Coconut Balls

Makes 12 servings

Prep. 12 minutes

Vegan, gluten-free

Rich and fruity, these convenient snacks are a taste sensation! The mango is high in vitamins C and A and contains the powerful antioxidant zeaxanthin, which has several health benefits. The coconut and pumpkin seeds are rich in healthy unsaturated fats, which can help to lower cholesterol. Like many of the snack balls in this book, these are Fuel dominant and therefore great to eat around training.

200g pitted dried dates, chopped

150g (1 ½ cups) porridge oats

75g frozen mango chunks, thawed (or use fresh mango)

50g pumpkin seeds

2 tbsp desiccated coconut

1 tsp coconut oil

1 tsp ground cinnamon

1. Soak the dates in boiling water for 1 minute. Drain in a colander.

2. Put the dates and the remaining ingredients in a food processor or blender and blitz until smooth.

3. Divide and roll into 12 balls. Leave to set in the fridge for at least 1 hour or until firm. Serve.

Nutrition: Heath score 1.8

Kcal	Carbs	Sugar	Protein	Fat	Sat Fat	Fibre
114.3	14.5g	8g (8.8%)	2.8g	4.5g	0.9g (4.5%)	2.7g (8.9%)

Apricot and Dark Chocolate Fuel Bars

Makes 10 servings

Prep. 15 minutes

Vegetarian, gluten-free

These delicious bars are called energy bars for a reason: they provide a good dose of carbs and are calorie dense; however, they have more protein and Health than your average energy bar. The pumpkin seeds and almonds provide minerals and healthy fats, and dark chocolate, which is rich in flavonoids, offers several health benefits, such as boosting brain and heart health and lowering cholesterol. The bars store really well, so make a batch and pop a bar into your exercise bag when needed over the next few weeks.

150g (1 ½ cups) porridge oats

70g pumpkin seeds

130g blanched almonds, chopped

75g dried apricots, chopped

100g golden syrup

100g clear honey

1 tbsp vanilla extract

100g chocolate, at least 85% cocoa solids, broken roughly

1. Put the oats in a mixing bowl and add the seeds, almonds and apricots.

2. Put the syrup and honey in a small saucepan over a medium heat and bring to the boil.

3. Stir in the vanilla, then pour into the mixing bowl with the oat mixture. Stir well.

4. Pour onto a baking sheet and spread evenly until about 1.5cm thick. Put in the fridge for 30 minutes. Once set, peel off the baking sheet.

5. Melt the chocolate in a heatproof bowl over a pan of gently simmering water, making sure that the base of the bowl doesn't touch the water. (Alternatively, use a microwave.) Trickle the chocolate over the seed mixture in a zigzag fashion. Cut into 10 bars.

Nutrition: Health score 3.2 High in vitamins B2, E and copper

Kcal	Carbs	Sugar	Protein	Fat	Sat Fat	Fibre
318.5	34g	21.6g (24%)	6.9g	16.2g	5.3g (26.5%)	5.1g (16.9%)

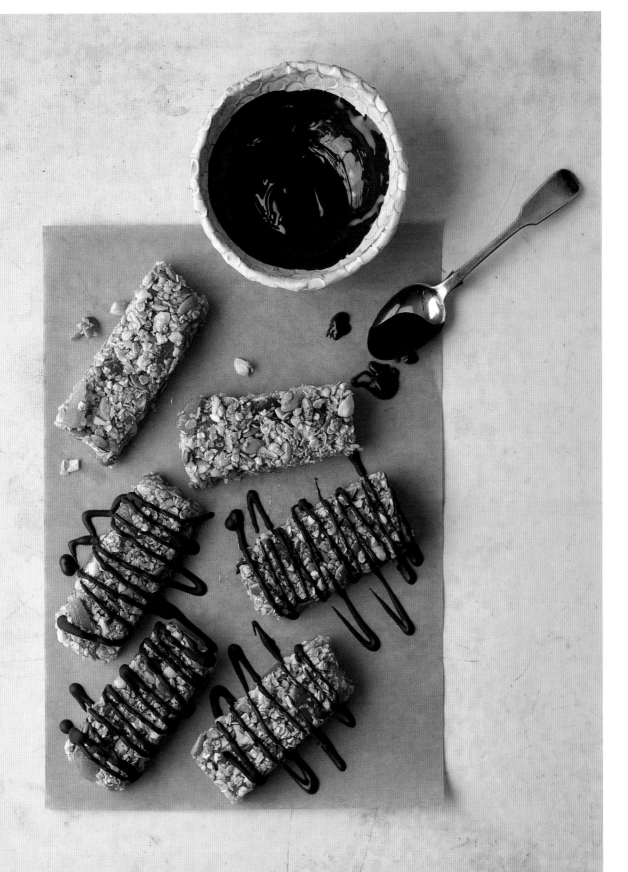

Walnut Chocolate Truffles

Makes 18 servings

Prep. 8 minutes

Vegan, gluten-free

Truffles are pure indulgence, surely? This version, however, has all the taste and texture of usual truffles, but with the benefits of dates and oats, which are packed full of fibre for a healthy digestive system. Cocoa is high in antioxidants and, along with the almond butter, it provides healthy monounsaturated fats. These truffles are a tasty Fuel choice for training – and a treat at any time.

200g pitted dried dates, chopped

100g walnuts

50g (½ cup) porridge oats

2 tbsp cocoa powder

100g almond butter

1. Soak the dates in boiling water for 15 minutes. Drain in a colander.
2. Put all the dry ingredients into a food processor and blitz until almost smooth. Tip into a bowl.
3. Put the dates in the food processor and blitz until smooth, then pour into the dry mixture.
4. Add the almond butter and mix well, using your hands. Divide and roll into 18 balls. Serve.

Nutrition: Health score 1.2 High in vitamin E, magnesium, potassium and manganese

Kcal	Carbs	Sugar	Protein	Fat	Sat Fat	Fibre
113.2	10.1g	7.5g (8.3%)	2.7g	7g	0.7g (3.3%)	2.3g (6%)

Apple, Oat and Mixed Seed Bars

Makes 8 servings

Prep. 10 minutes

Vegan, gluten-free

Speedy to make, these delicious apple snack bars will be popular with all the family, plus they're healthy, unlike most of the bars you buy. The oats make a great low-glycaemic base (see page 221), and the seeds provide healthy unsaturated fats, plus they are high in minerals such as iron.

300g (3 cups) porridge oats

4 tbsp mixed seeds

150g apple sauce from a jar

55g reduced-fat margarine or vegan alternative

1. Preheat the oven to 200°C (180°C fan oven) Gas 6. Put the oats and seeds in a large mixing bowl.

2. Heat the apple sauce and margarine in a small saucepan over a medium heat until dissolved.

3. Whisk the apple mixture until smooth, then pour it over the oats. Stir well, then pack into a small traybake tin or baking tray. Bake for 15–20 minutes until golden. Score into eight bars while still hot, then leave to cool completely. Cut into bars and serve.

Nutrition: Health score 2.6 High in vitamin B1, copper and manganese

Kcal	Carbs	Sugar	Protein	Fat	Sat Fat	Fibre
224.2	24g	2.3g (2.5%)	6.1g	10.1g	1.7g (8.5%)	4.3g (14.5%)

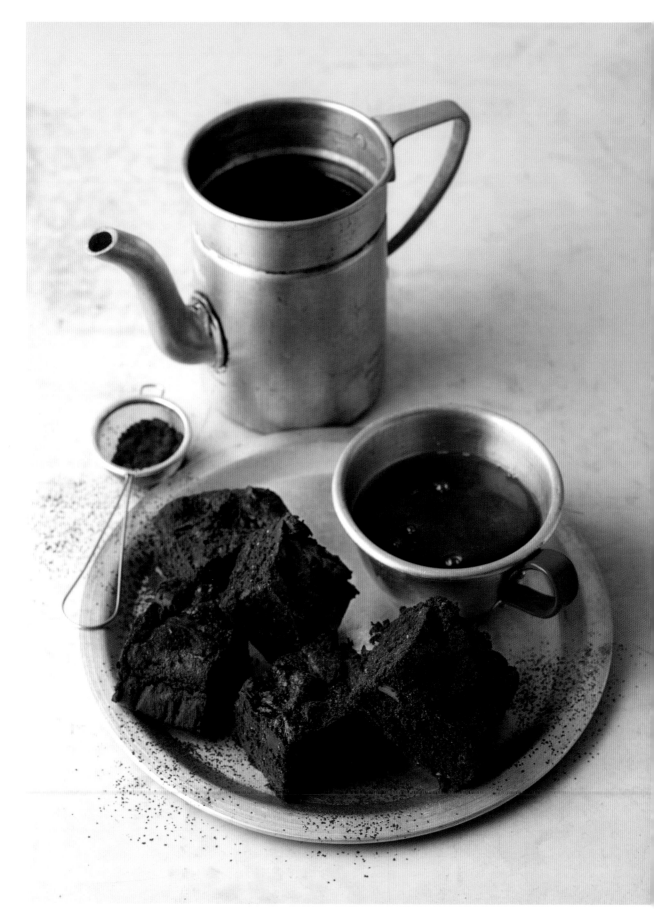

Avocado Brownies

Makes 10 servings

Prep. 12 minutes

Vegetarian

How can a brownie be healthy? Simply by using healthy ingredients. Cocoa powder and dark chocolate are high in antioxidants and healthy fat, and avocado is high in healthy monounsaturated fat and several vitamins and minerals. You can enjoy a brownie with a clear conscious when you have your cup of tea.

100g honey

1 tsp vanilla extract

100ml milk

2 eggs

1 large avocado, halved, pitted and flesh scooped

75g (½ cup) plain wholemeal flour

30g cocoa powder

1 tsp baking powder

100g dark chocolate, broken roughly into small pieces

1. Preheat the oven to 190°C (170°C fan oven) Gas 5, and line a 20 x 20cm traybake tin with baking paper. Put all the wet ingredients into a food processor or blender and blitz until smooth.

2. Mix the flour, cocoa and baking powder in a bowl, then slowly fold in the blended liquid. Pour the batter into the prepared tin and smooth it out evenly. Push the broken chocolate pieces into the top of the mixture.

3. Bake for 20–25 minutes until firm. Cool and cut into 10 squares. Serve.

Nutrition: Health score 2 High in copper and iron

Kcal	Carbs	Sugar	Protein	Fat	Sat Fat	Fibre
165.3	18.1g	11.4g (12.7%)	3.9g	8.1g	3.4g (17.1%)	3.2g (12.7%)

Banana and Date Flapjacks

Makes 6 servings

Prep. 12 minutes

Vegetarian, gluten-free

With a few natural additions, flapjacks can be healthy and extremely tasty – leaving you longing for more. The dates and bananas add a wonderful gooey texture, plus they contain minerals such as potassium. This is very much a fuel-based snack, and so it is perfect to eat around exercise.

110g pitted dried dates, chopped

50g ground almonds

2 bananas

2 tbsp honey

1 tsp ground cinnamon

100g (1 cup) porridge oats

1. Preheat the oven to 200°C (180°C fan oven) Gas 6. Put the dates in a bowl and cover with boiling water. Leave to soak for 1 minute.

2. Put the almonds in a food processor or blender and add the bananas, honey, cinnamon and 50ml water. Blitz until smooth.

3. Put the oats in a bowl and pour the banana mixture over the top. Mix thoroughly to combine.

4. Spread the mixture onto a baking tray until about 1.5cm thick. Bake for 15 minutes.

5. Score into 6 bars while hot, then leave to cool. Cut into bars when cold. Serve.

Nutrition: Health score 1.5 High in vitamins B2, B6 and E

Kcal	Carbs	Sugar	Protein	Fat	Sat Fat	Fibre
213.3	35.9g	21.7g (24.1%)	4.4g	5.5g	0.5g (2.7%)	5g (16.8%)

Fig, Hazelnut and Dark Chocolate Bars

Makes 6 servings

Prep. 10 minutes

Vegan, gluten-free

Perhaps surprisingly, these chocolate bars are crammed full of health benefits! Figs are a great source of minerals, including potassium and copper, and hazelnuts are rich in magnesium and healthy unsaturated fats. The bars have quite a high sugar content, so it's best to eat them mainly around exercise, but once you taste them, you will want them all the time.

50g dark chocolate, at least 85% cocoa solids, broken roughly

100g pitted dried dates, chopped

150g dried figs, chopped

60g hazelnuts

100g (1 cup) porridge oats

1. Melt the chocolate in a heatproof bowl over a pan of gently simmering water, making sure that the base of the bowl doesn't touch the water. (Alternatively, use a microwave.)

2. Soak the dates and figs in a bowl with boiling water for 1 minute. Drain in a colander.

3. Put the hazelnuts in a food processor, then blitz to make a fine powder. Add the oats, dates and figs, and blitz until smooth.

4. Add the mixture to the melted chocolate and stir to combine well.

5. Spoon the mixture into a six-cup cake tin. Put in the fridge for at least 1 hour or until firm. Serve.

Nutrition: Health Score 3.1. High in copper, potassium and manganese

Kcal	Carbs	Sugar	Protein	Fat	Sat Fat	Fibre
282.4	38.4g	25.2g (28%)	5.1g	11.1g	2.7g (13.5%)	7g (18.5%)

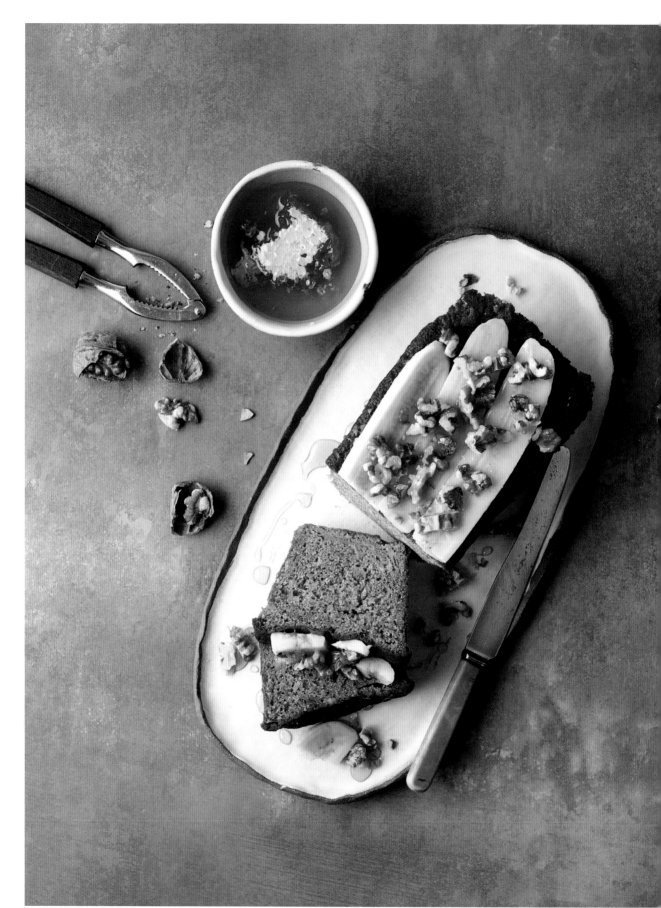

Banana Bread

Serves 10

Prep. 18 minutes

Vegetarian

For me, one slice of this bread is never enough, although all that taste does come at a slight cost. It is reasonably high in sugar, and therefore calories, but that's not usual for a snack. The bananas, walnuts and cinnamon all have health benefits, however, making it better than most bought sweet snack options. It's a perfect snack when you are going to be involved in a high-energy-expenditure activity or sport.

150g butter, softened

150g (¾ cup) caster sugar

2 eggs

150g (generous 1 cup) self-raising flour

1 tsp baking powder

1 tbsp ground cinnamon

2 bananas

sliced banana, chopped walnuts and honey, to decorate

1. Preheat the oven to 180°C (160°C fan oven) Gas 4 and line a 900g loaf tin with baking paper. In a mixing bowl, beat together the butter and sugar using a wooden spoon or electric beater.

2. Beat in 1 egg, then sift in some of the flour, the baking powder and cinnamon. Beat in the other egg. Mash the bananas and stir in.

3. Sift in the remaining flour and stir well to combine. Spoon into the tin and level the top. Bake for 55 minutes or until firm to the touch and golden. Cool in the tin, then turn out.

4. Decorate with slices of banana, walnuts and a drizzle of honey.

Nutrition: Health score 1.8 High in vitamins B1, B2 and A

Kcal	Carbs	Sugar	Protein	Fat	Sat Fat	Fibre
289.5	33.7g	20.6g (22.9%)	3.6g	16g	8.2g (40.8%)	1.7g (14.5%)

Blueberry and Banana Oat Muffins

Serves 12

Prep. 15 minutes

Vegetarian

Oats make these muffins particularly healthy, combined with the fruit, and they are a real winner with the kids. They are high in carbs, but the oat base means that the energy is released more slowly, meaning that your insulin levels and blood glucose remain more stable. The eggs add some protein, and blueberries have really high antioxidant properties. Be careful when you make a batch, though, you'll want to eat them all!

50g butter

100g (¾ cup) self-raising flour

1 tbsp baking powder

100g (1 cup) porridge oats

50g (¼ cup) caster sugar

3 eggs

1 banana

250ml milk

100g frozen blueberries

1. Preheat the oven to 190°C (170°C fan oven) Gas 5. Put 12 muffin cases in a muffin tray or on a baking tray. Melt the butter in a small saucepan over a medium heat.

2. Sift the flour and baking powder into a large mixing bowl and add the oats and sugar.

3. Beat the eggs in a bowl, then slowly add the melted butter and mix in.

4. Mash the banana. Add the butter mixture to the oat mixture, then add the milk and banana. Stir to combine but don't over-mix. Gently stir in the blueberries.

5. Spoon the mixture into the muffin cases and bake for 30 minutes or until firm to the touch. Cool completely.

Nutrition: Health score 1.2 High in vitamins A and D

Kcal	Carbs	Sugar	Protein	Fat	Sat Fat	Fibre
146.2	18.9g	7.7g (8.5%)	4.2g	5.8g	2.9g (14.3%)	2g (5.4%)

Joint Panna Cotta

Serves 3

Prep. 12 minutes

Gluten-free

This low-calorie panna cotta tastes amazing and is designed to support and strengthen the tendons and ligaments by using gelatin and vitamin C to promote collagen production. Optimally, consume it around 30 minutes before exercise or rehabilitation to ensure that the collagen reaches the targeted ligaments. Collagen is also great for our skin health.

200ml milk

2 gelatine sheets

20g (1 scoop) vanilla protein powder

2 tbsp low-fat Greek yogurt

1. Heat the milk in a saucepan over a medium heat until boiling. Take the milk off the heat and add the gelatine. Stir until thickened.

2. Add the protein powder and whisk until fully combined.

3. Leave for 5–10 minutes or until cooled, then add the yogurt and whisk until fully combined.

4. Pour the mixture into 3 ramekins and chill in the fridge for 1 hour before serving.

Nutrition: Health score 1.8 High in copper, potassium and manganese

Kcal	Carbs	Sugar	Protein	Fat	Sat Fat	Fibre
93.2	4g	4.2g (4.7%)	13g	2.7g	1.4g (7.2%)	0.2g (0.4%)

Healthy Eton Mess

Serves 1

Prep. 4 minutes

Vegan

My healthy slant on the classic dessert uses granola to provide crunch, instead of having meringue, making it lower in sugar and higher in fibre than the standard version. I have substituted Greek yogurt for the ice cream and cream because it's lower in fat and higher in protein. The mixed berries provide lots of flavour and are high in vitamin C. Although not quite like the real thing, it's a super-quick, no-guilt treat that my kids absolutely love for breakfast or as a snack.

70g frozen berries, thawed or microwaved for 1 minute

5 tbsp Greek yogurt, or vegan alternative

½ tsp vanilla extract

2 tbsp granola

1. Put the berries in a bowl and lightly mash them using a fork.
2. Add the remaining ingredients and mix through. Serve.

Nutrition: Health score 1.7 High in vitamins B2, B12 and manganese

Kcal	Carbs	Sugar	Protein	Fat	Sat Fat	Fibre
151.4	17.3g	12.3g (13.6%)	9.8g	3.5g	1.1g (5.7%)	2.5g (8.2%)

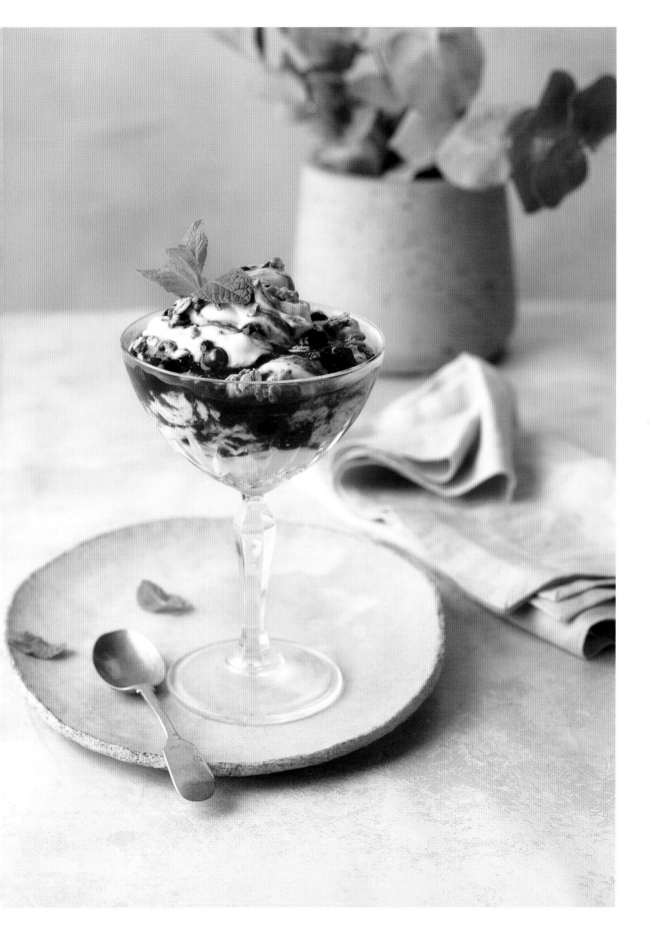

Balls Builder

Energy balls and protein balls have become in vogue of late as a convenient snack that is associated with healthy snacking and training. Here's how to put together your own version.

- The key to making balls is a binding agent to keep them all together. The binding agent is normally some form of dried fruit, with dates being very popular. I recommend soaking dried fruit in boiling water for about 1 minute, so that they blend more easily.

- Adding a further binding agent is common, although not always necessary if you have used dates. Almond butter, avocado and coconut oil are good binding agents and will add healthy fats, but they will also increase the calorie hit.

- Oats and/or nuts and seeds normally form the base ingredient, providing Fuel and some protein. Fruit adds health benefits but dried fruit does have high sugar levels.

- If you want to increase Lean Muscle content, protein powders are commonly used, as they bind well and can add to the flavour. Other so-called superfood powders, such as spirulina and maca, add a further healthy element but might detract from the flavour.

- Pop all the ingredients into a blender to chop and blend well.

- Put oil on your hands to help prevent sticking and then shape the balls. You can then coat them for appearance, taste and health purposes. Cocoa and desiccated coconut are popular coatings.

PERFORMANCE
FUEL

LEAN
MUSCLE

HEALTH

Ingredients

Nuts, seeds, oats 100g	Fruit ~ 200g	Powder 1-2 tsp	Sticky stuff ~ 1 tbsp	Coatings Variable
Almond, cashew	Dates, figs	Protein	Peanut, almond butter	Chia seeds
Walnut, pecan	Apricots	 Acai, maca	Honey	Cocoa, cinnamon
Pumpkins, flax, chia	Goji, raisin, cranberry	Cocoa powder	Coconut oil	Desiccated coconut
Oats	Soft fruit	Spirulina	Sticky fruit	Crushed nuts

Method

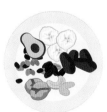

1. Ingredients
Place all ingredients together in the bowl of a food processor

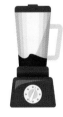

2. Whizz it up
Whizz all ingredients until they bind together to form a stiff paste

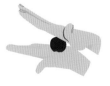

3. Get rolling
Divide the mixture into evenly sized balls and place on a tray or plate

4. Cover it up
Spread your coating evenly on a separate plate or dish and roll the balls in it

5. Leave to set
Place the balls in the fridge for 1 hour to help set them

SMOOTHIES

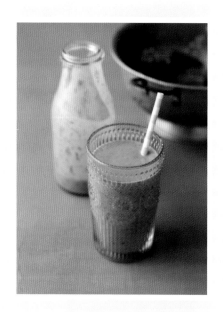

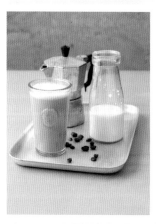

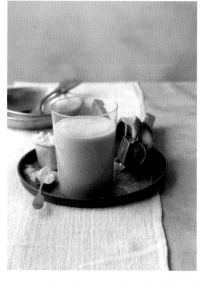

Pear and Apple Smoothie

Serves 1

Prep. 2 minutes

Vegan, gluten-free

This refreshing green smoothie packs a serious health kick: the vitamins reel off like the alphabet. It has half the recommended daily allowance (RDA) for vitamins C and K, calcium, phosphorus and potassium, and well over 100 per cent RDA for vitamin A, which helps you to fight disease and feel great. It is quite a rounded smoothie, but it is Fuel dominant, so it will be a good choice when you are active.

1 pear, cored

1 apple, cored

75g green grapes

2 handfuls of baby spinach

200ml milk, or vegan alternative

20g (1 scoop) vanilla protein powder, or vegan alternative

Put all the ingredients into a food processor or blender and blitz until smooth. Serve.

Nutrition: Health score 10.3 High in vitamins B2, B12, A, C and K

Kcal	Carbs	Sugar	Protein	Fat	Sat Fat	Fibre
472	71.7g	62.3g (69.2%)	27g	6.4g	3.7g (18.4%)	12g (31.6%)

Post-Workout Peanut Butter Blast

Serves 1

Prep. 2 minutes

Vegan, gluten-free

Tasty, thick and creamy, this nutty smoothie is packed with protein. In fact, it contains all three macronutrients to provide the perfect blend of recovery ingredients after your workout. High in plant foods, it counts as three of your five-a-day, providing a whole host of micronutrients to support your health. It has a fairly high calorie load, so it is a good choice for those wishing to put on muscle mass.

a handful of kale

½ banana

small apple

1 tbsp peanut butter

20g (1 scoop) protein powder, or vegan alternative

375ml almond milk

Put all the ingredients into a food processor or blender and blitz until smooth. Serve.

Nutrition: Health score 7.1 High in vitamins B2, B5, C and D, copper and calcium

Kcal	Carbs	Sugar	Protein	Fat	Sat Fat	Fibre
412.2	38.5g	28.6g (31.8%)	31g	13.8g	2.1g (10.7%)	6.5g (17.1%)

Beetroot and Mixed Berry Smoothie

Serves 1

Prep. 2 minutes

Vegan, gluten-free

This smoothie will set you up for peak performance. The nitrates in beetroot shots act as a vasodilator, which means that you can supply more blood and oxygen to your muscles and organs. As an added bonus, it's also anti-ageing. The berries add a good amount of vitamin C and the banana is a great fuel source for exercise and contains potassium to aid muscle stimulation.

1 banana

250g natural yogurt, or vegan alternative

130g frozen mixed berries

a handful of ice cubes

250ml water

70ml ready-made beetroot shot

Put all the ingredients into a food processor or blender and blitz until smooth. Serve.

Nutrition: Health score 2.5 High in vitamins B2, B5, A and C

Kcal	Carbs	Sugar	Protein	Fat	Sat Fat	Fibre
216.2	35.9g	28.2g (31.3%)	6.9g	4.2g	2.6g (13.2%)	3.8g (10%)

Creamy Dream Smoothie

Serves 1

Prep. 3 minutes

Vegan, gluten-free

250ml almond milk

20g (1 scoop) protein powder,
or vegan alternative

½ avocado

a handful of baby spinach

½ banana

5 ice cubes

This creamy smoothie is a taste sensation, with a high health score from its range of vitamins, minerals and good fats. It is reasonably calorie dense because it contains avocado and banana, but its high protein content means that it staves off hunger for some time and it can function well as a post-workout shake.

Put all the ingredients into a food processor or blender and blitz until smooth. Serve.

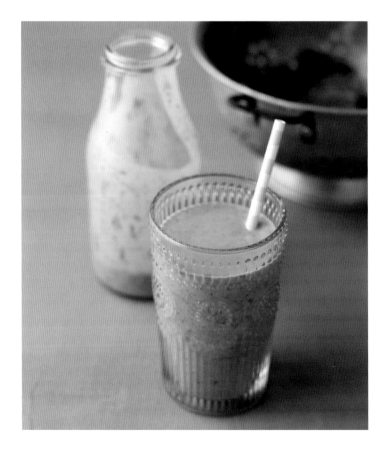

Nutrition: Health score 7.0 High in vitamins B2, B5, A and D, K and calcium

Kcal	Carbs	Sugar	Protein	Fat	Sat Fat	Fibre
332.9	18.9g	11.4g (12.7%)	27.8g	14.4g	1.9g (9.5%)	6.8g (17.9%)

Protein Frappuccino

Serves 1

Prep. 2 minutes

Vegan, gluten-free

The almond milk and protein powder in this delicious iced smoothie provide vitamins A, D and E, which help us to look good, and the high protein content will help us to stay lean. The caffeine also provides a little pick-me-up. What better way to cool down on a hot day?

250ml almond milk

20g (1 scoop) vanilla whey protein powder, or vegan alternative

a handful of ice cubes

250ml brewed coffee

Put all the ingredients into a food processor or blender and blitz until smooth. Serve.

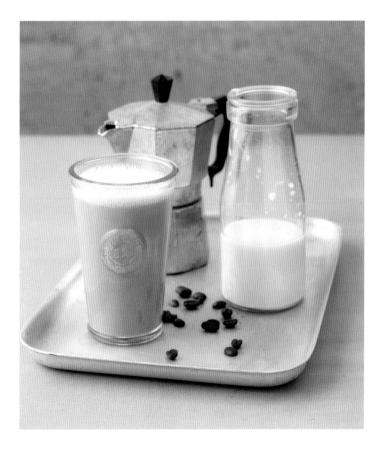

Nutrition: Health score 2.9 High in vitamins B2, B5, A and D

Kcal	Carbs	Sugar	Protein	Fat	Sat Fat	Fibre
165.9	5.3g	3.9g (4.3%)	25.7g	3.7g	0.4g (1.9%)	2.8g (7.3%)

Lean Strawberry Smoothie

Serves 1

Prep. 1 minute

Vegan, gluten-free

Sweet strawberries give this smoothie lots of flavour, and it also packs a big protein punch thanks to the Greek yogurt and protein powder. In fact, it's a nutritional powerhouse, full of B vitamins, vitamins A, C and D, and a range of minerals to help you stay in peak health. Give it a go for breakfast or as a great muscle-boosting snack.

100g strawberries

200ml milk, or vegan alternative

200ml Greek yogurt, or vegan alternative

20g (1 scoop) strawberry or vanilla protein powder, or vegan alternative

Put all the ingredients into a food processor or blender and blitz until smooth. Serve.

Nutrition: Health score 5.9 High in vitamins B2 and C

Kcal	Carbs	Sugar	Protein	Fat	Sat Fat	Fibre
412.6	29.3g	27.9g (31%)	51.2g	8.7g	4.3g (21.7%)	3g (10.1%)

Berry Booster Smoothie

Serves 1

Prep. 1 minute

Vegan, gluten-free

60g mixed berries, fresh or frozen

100ml semi-skimmed milk, or vegan alternative

4 scoops Greek yogurt, or vegan alternative

a very small handful of baby spinach

Smoothies using berries are always popular. A classic made with ingredients you probably have to hand. It is reasonably balanced with the Greek yogurt and milk providing some protein, but the berries make it Fuel and Health dominant.

Put all the ingredients into a food processor or blender and blitz until smooth. Serve.

Nutrition: Health score 5.2 High in vitamins A, B12 and K

Kcal	Carbs	Sugar	Protein	Fat	Sat Fat	Fibre
161.3	21.2g	17.7g (19.7%)	11.6g	2.2g	1.2g (6%)	3.8g (12.5%)

Almond and Ginger Smoothie

Serves 1

Prep. 2 minutes

Vegan, gluten-free

200ml almond milk

1cm fresh ginger, peeled

2 tbsp almond butter

½ banana

2 tbsp linseeds

Full of health benefits, this ginger-based smoothie will help you to look and feel great. Ginger is a powerful antioxidant and anti-inflammatory, in addition to adding its unique taste and warmth to the mix.

Put all the ingredients into a food processor or blender and blitz until smooth. Serve.

Nutrition: Health score 7.3 High in vitamin E, calcium and copper

Kcal	Carbs	Sugar	Protein	Fat	Sat Fat	Fibre
354.6	17.1g	8.9g (9.9%)	11.1g	25.7g	1.9g (9.4%)	8.7g (29%)

Mango and Orange Smoothie

Serves 1

Prep. 2 minutes

Vegan, gluten-free

Wildly fruity, this smoothie is a real crowd-pleaser as it looks and tastes amazing. Orange and mango are both high in vitamin C, and orange plant foods also contain beta-carotene – both those nutrients support your immune system. Orange juice is a little high in sugar, but you can swap it for water if you like. The high levels of potassium and carbs make this a great choice if you're going to be active.

1 mango, or 175g frozen mango

150ml orange juice

20g (1 scoop) vanilla protein powder, or vegan alternative

Using a sharp knife, cut each side of the mango away from the large pit in the centre. Score rough squares into the mango flesh and then push the skin side inwards to make the mango cubes stand proud. Cut off the cubes. Cut off the flesh around the pit. Put all the ingredients into a food processor or blender and blitz until smooth. Serve.

Nutrition: Health score 5.8 High in vitamins A, C and copper

Kcal	Carbs	Sugar	Protein	Fat	Sat Fat	Fibre
277.6	50g	44.1g (49%)	17.5g	1.6g	0.5g (2.3%)	5.4g (14.1%)

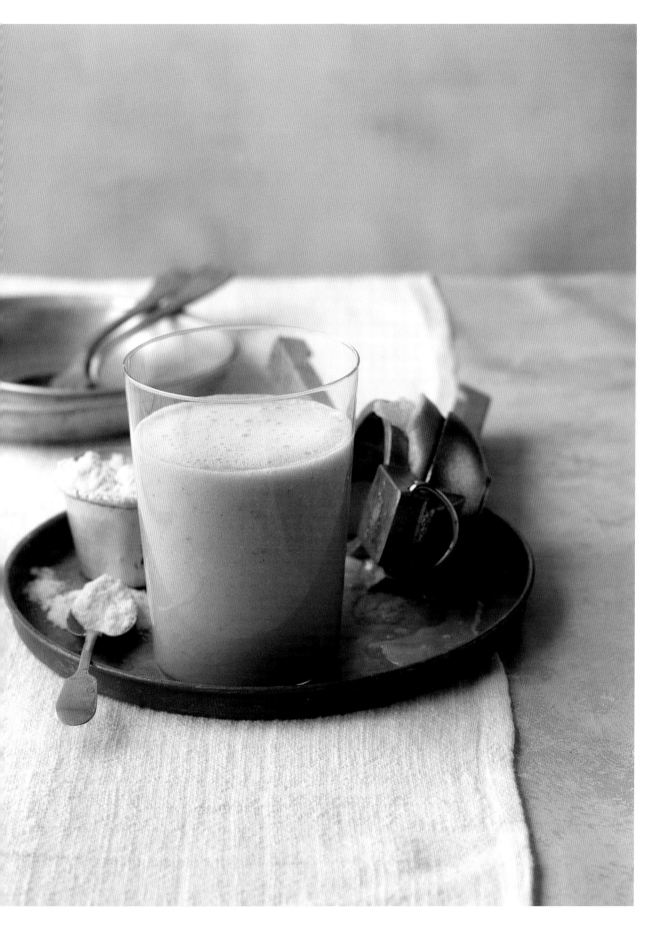

Smoothie Builder

Smoothies are extremely popular, and rightly so. They are so quick, tasty and packed full of health benefits. People often view them as something that they just add to their existing diet but most smoothies can be quite calorific and high in sugars, so they should be viewed as a meal or snack. Get creative and try making your own concoctions with this simple guide.

- We *drink* smoothies, so liquid is the foundation. Water is normally fine, as we get the nutrition from other elements. For taste or to increase Lean Muscle content you can use milk. As a post-workout smoothie, milk is great, as it provides slow-release casein proteins to work in tandem with the fast-release protein from protein powders, in addition to adding natural electrolytes to help hydration.

- To increase Lean Muscle, protein powders are convenient and add flavour. High-protein yogurt can be used and provides a nice creamy texture.

- Fruit adds Health and Fuel, in addition to a great taste. Berries are very popular, as you don't have to chop them and they are relatively low in sugar. Frozen fruit works well to keep costs down and makes a nice cool drink.

- The Health element can be increased with some leafy greens, such as spinach or kale.

- Healthy fats can be obtained from avocado, nut butters, nuts and seeds, but they will ramp up the calories.

- The finishing touch can be a healthy flavouring such as cinnamon, especially if you have included a lot of leafy greens, but the beauty of smoothies is that they are normally delicious already.

- Whip them all up in a blender and your smoothie is ready in seconds.

PERFORMANCE
FUEL

LEAN
MUSCLE

HEALTH

1. Choose your base

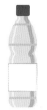
Water

Animal or
nut milk

Coconut
water

Ice cubes

2. Add your protein

Protein
powder

Milk

Greek yogurt

3. Prepare the fruit

Mango

Apple

Berries

Watermelon

Orange

Grapes

Peach

Pineapple

Banana

Cherry

Pear

Kiwi

4. Add your greens

Spinach

Kale

Swiss chard

Watercress

5. Add healthy fats

Avocado

Nuts

Nut butter

Seeds

6. Supercharge with extras

Manuka
honey

Cinnamon

Cacoa
powder

Maca
powder

PART 2
COLOUR-FIT TRAINING

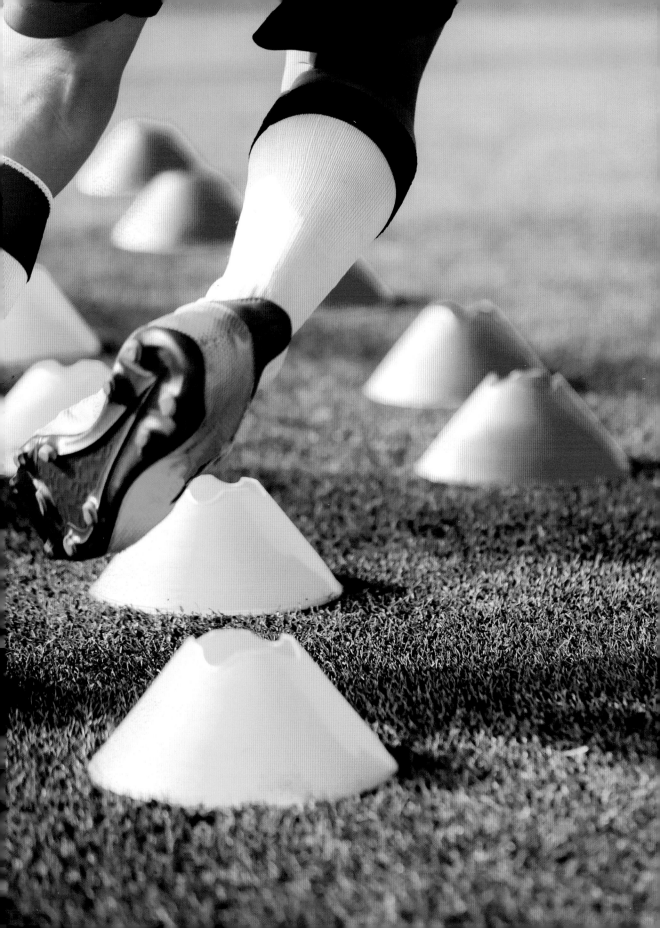

Colour-Fit Cook shows us how to eat to achieve our goals, but if you want to achieve optimal results – be it a health, fitness or appearance goal – you should also perform appropriate training. Thankfully, Colour-Fit was born in professional training and our team contains world-leading experts from numerous fitness and sport backgrounds, so you're in great hands. The training principles – and plans in Part 3 – apply to any level of training, so it doesn't matter if you are preparing for your first parkrun or want to smash an Olympic triathlon, reduce your waistline or improve your health, Colour-Fit Training can help.

Colour-Fit Training Methods

In accordance with Colour-Fit's founding principle of making things simple, the team and I have re-shaped the way most people look at training to make it more intuitive. We have categorised different training methods in relation to the training goal or description to make selecting appropriate training methods as simple as possible. Furthermore, we invented Colour-Fit Training Load Gauges, which allow you to gauge easily what types of training you will be doing and how hard the training is going to be. I will expand more on the Training Load Gauges in the Training Plan section.

Endurance and strength training form the foundations from which we attain the majority of our training goals, be it for performance, body shape or health, so let's explore the evidence base behind the Colour-Fit approach to endurance and strength training. Understanding this will allow you to follow our training programmes easily and to adapt and build your own programmes to match your unique lifestyle and goals.

Endurance training

Endurance training is the cornerstone of popular activities such as running and cycling, in addition to prolonged sports such as football, rugby and tennis. Most of us who go to the gym perform some form of endurance on the varied CV (cardiovascular) machines and in fitness classes. Endurance training is the foundation of getting generally fitter, healthier and leaner, and it is recommended that all of us should perform some form of endurance training regularly.

Endurance is classically associated with lower intensity, longer duration efforts, but it can also involve a range of intensities right up to maximum efforts that are repeated. The energy required to perform endurance training is generated from our two energy systems – the aerobic system and the anaerobic system – which are recruited differentially dependent on the intensity and duration of the exercise.

The aerobic system requires oxygen to produce energy and is therefore heavily reliant on the heart and lungs to work harder when we exercise to transport extra oxygen to our muscles where it is used to create energy. It can produce only moderate amounts of energy but can do so for long periods and is therefore critical in longer events such as marathons.

The anaerobic system can produce high levels of energy very quickly, without the need for oxygen. It can only do so over short periods – about 10 seconds if exercise is maximal and 1–2 minutes if the exercise is near maximal – as it produces several fatigue inducing by-products, such as acids. The anaerobic system is key to shorter, high-intensity events, such as sprints.

If we gradually increase exercise intensity, anaerobic energy contribution will begin at moderate levels, known as the 'aerobic threshold'. Levels of the fatiguing metabolites increase, but very gradually because we are able to clear them nearly as fast as they are produced, therefore we do not fatigue and can continue exercising. As intensity increases further, we reach a point where the fatiguing by-products rise exponentially as we become unable to clear them sufficiently, forcing us to slow down or stop. The point just before this exponential rise is known as 'anaerobic threshold' and represents the highest intensity we can exercise for a sustained period.

EXERCISE INTENSITY

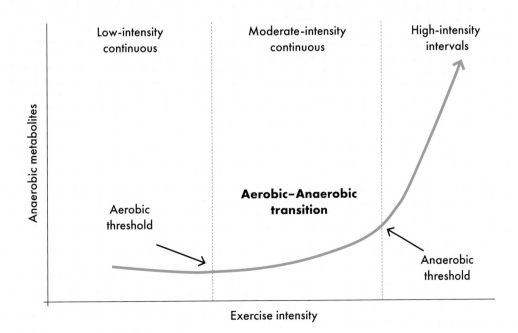

Colour-Fit endurance training uses these key points in anaerobic energy contribution to control the length of time we can train before fatiguing. Controlling and optimising training intensity and duration means that we can target specific training goals, such as boosting an energy system that is important to performance in a specific sport or maximising calorie burn in order to become lean. Below we discuss the different Colour-Fit endurance training categories and how best to perform them to attain your chosen goals.

Categories of Colour-Fit endurance training

Steady Endurance is classic endurance training, where you train at a *steady* pace for a relatively extensive period. It involves low-to-moderate intensity exercise around aerobic threshold up to slightly below anaerobic threshold, where breathing is increased but remains steady. Exercise durations can vary massively depending on your fitness, but extensive would normally mean over about 20 minutes although it can go on for hours. The extensive use and predominance of the aerobic system during this training makes it more efficient so that we can exercise for longer. Therefore, it is suited for sports where exercise duration can be extensive, such as running, cycling, swimming and prolonged sports such as football and rugby.

The reliance of the aerobic system on the heart, lungs and blood to deliver oxygen means that health markers such as heart function and blood pressure are improved and it is therefore suitable for those wanting to improve their general health and fitness. The extensive nature also means that we can potentially burn lots of calories, and the moderate intensity means that we are able to use a greater proportion of fat for energy, which is great for weight maintenance or weight loss.

Threshold Endurance involves training at a pace close to the anaerobic *threshold*. It is a moderate-to-hard intensity that is the *threshold* of being uncomfortable. The anaerobic threshold is the highest point of aerobic stress that we can tolerate for an extensive period, which results in adaptations that make us faster over prolonged periods. Therefore, threshold training is suited to those who want to improve their endurance performance, especially over moderate durations (20–60 minutes; for example, 5–10km runs), but it is also suitable for anyone wanting to improve their general health and fitness.

Appropriate intensities can be gauged by exercising as hard as possible for 15–20 minutes (15 minutes for lower fitness and 20 minutes for high fitness). For example, a cyclist who managed to cover 10km in 15 minutes would have a threshold speed of approximately 667m/min or could use average watts. More simply, you can estimate threshold intensity by pushing to the point where your breathing goes from steady to quick but is not ever-increasing and exercise feels quite hard. Appropriate exercise durations normally range from 10–30 minutes over one or multiple repetitions (reps), but elite endurance athletes can complete marathons at this pace, so if you are really fit you can go for longer.

Maximal Aerobic Endurance involves training at the cusp of where the *aerobic* system is working *maximally*. This is a fast pace where the anaerobic system is used to the extent that it causes fatigue. Therefore, intervals are used to prolong the total training time. Because it is the lowest intensity of working the aerobic system maximally, we can expose the aerobic system to a maximal stimulus for as long as possible. As such, maximal aerobic training is a powerful stimulus for aerobic adaptations that improve both longer and more intense endurance activities. It is a popular training method for most endurance events and in sports where you work at a range of intensities (for example, basketball and football).

The appropriate pace can be gauged by exercising maximally for 4–5 minutes (4 minutes for lower fitness and 5 minutes for high fitness) and using the average speed/power. For example, a runner who covered 1100 metres in 4 minutes would have a maximal aerobic speed of approximately 275m/min or 4.6m/sec. Intervals are normally 2–5 minutes long, but can be as short as 30 seconds, and are repeated for a total of 10–20 minutes. Rest times between intervals are around half-to-equal work durations, so if you worked for 4 minutes a half rest time would be 2 minutes.

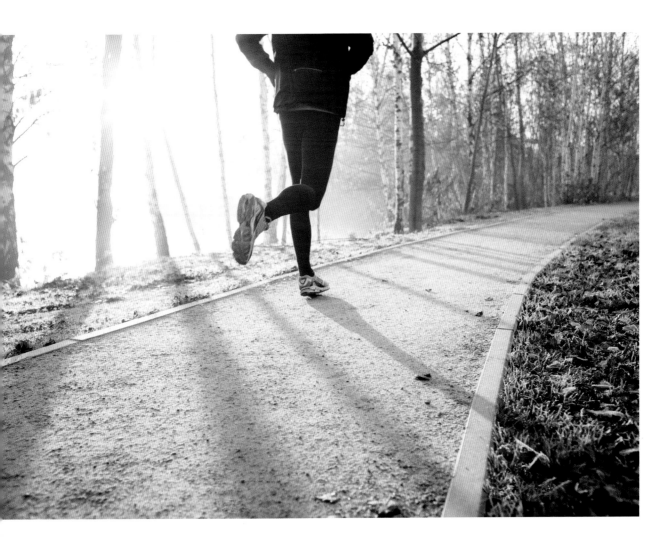

Maximal Interval Endurance involves *maximal* or near-maximal intensity efforts, that are performed over multiple *intervals*. Traditionally, such high intensities were avoided for endurance training because durations are short due to rapid fatigue; however, maximal intervals, or HIIT training, has become incredibly popular recently as a time-efficient form of enhancing not only anaerobic fitness but also aerobic fitness and weight management. Aerobic fitness is improved because the aerobic system is recruited maximally with each bout, and it restores important fast-acting anaerobic energy substrates (basically the molecules that help create energy in our cells) during the rest periods. High levels of anaerobic energy enhance this energy system, and the resultant high levels of fatiguing metabolites stimulate adaptations that hasten their removal.

These adaptations mean that we can exercise maximally for longer, which is important in many sports, but it also improves our anaerobic threshold pace, which is good for longer events. While overall metabolic cost is moderate due to the relatively short training duration, enhanced weight management is achieved through increased energy burning at rest. Appropriate intensities are fairly self-explanatory: you either go maximally or very close to it.

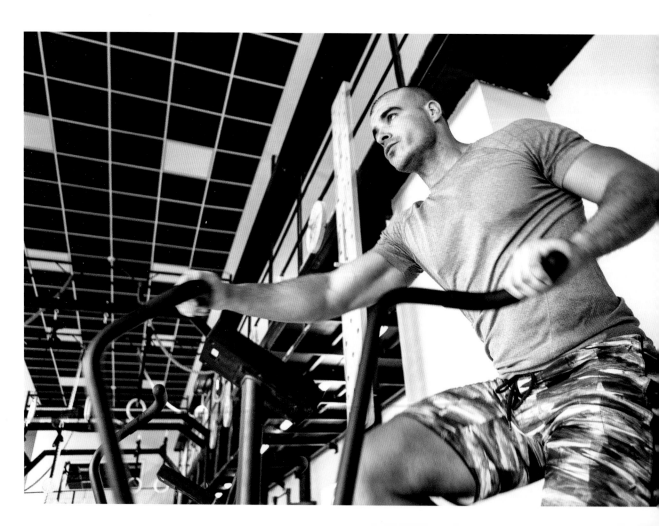

Protocols for maximal interval training vary considerably. Those at maximal pace normally last less than 10 seconds for multiple reps with rest periods longer than work periods. Those at near-maximal pace last about 20 seconds to 2 minutes and involve multiple reps with rest times less than work time when aerobic adaptations are desired, and longer rest periods when anaerobic adaptations take precedence. A popular example is Tabata intervals, which consist of repeated 20-second high-intensity efforts, separated by 10 seconds rest for about 4 minutes.

The tables below and overleaf highlight the Colour-Fit approach to different endurance training methods and typical training structures depending upon your level of fitness. The graph on the next page illustrates the relationship between exercise intensity and duration for the different training methods.

Abbreviations used in the tables		reps	repetitions
BP	blood pressure	~	approximately
CV	cardiovascular	>	greater than
HRmax	maximum heart rate	<	less than

BENEFITS AND STRUCTURE OUTLINE FOR THE ENDURANCE TRAINING METHODS

Method	Benefits	Effort/intensity	Structure
Steady	• Go longer/further • High calorie and fat burn • Healthy heart and BP	• Easy-to-moderate • Steady breathing • 60–80% HRmax	• Normally continuous or short rest • 20 minutes to several hours
Threshold	• Go faster for long periods • Calorie burn • Healthy heart and BP	• Moderate-to-hard • Fast but steady breathing • 15–20 minutes max pace • 80–90% HRmax	• Continuous or intervals with short rest • 20–60 minutes (normally <30 minutes) • Intervals > 5 minutes
Maximal aerobic	• Faster over long and shorter periods • Healthy heart and BP • Time efficient	• Hard • Heavy breathing • 4–5 minutes max pace • 90–95% HRmax	• 30 second–5 minute (normally > 2 minutes) intervals for total of 10–20 minutes • Rest: half–equal work time
Maximal intervals	• Work maximally for longer; recover quicker • Increased metabolism • Time efficient	• Near max–maximal • Heavy breathing	• Varied. 5–90 second intervals for 4–20 minutes • Rest: 0.5–5 ratio to work time

PROGRESSIVE STRUCTURES FOR ENDURANCE TRAINING METHODS BASED ON FITNESS LEVELS

Steady				
Level	Total duration	Rep. duration	Reps	Rest
Beginner	15–40 minutes	10–30 seconds	2–4	<2 minutes
Quite fit	30–60 minutes	10–60 seconds	2–6	<1 minute
Very fit	>60 minutes	n/a	1	n/a
Threshold				
Beginner	15–25 minutes	5–10 seconds	2–5	<2 minutes
Quite fit	20–30 minutes	8–15 seconds	2–6	<2 minutes
Very fit	>30 minutes	10–20 seconds	3–6	<2 minutes
Maximal aerobic				
Beginner	10–12 minutes	1–2 seconds	5–12	~ equal work time
Quite fit	12–16 minutes	2–4 seconds	4–8	½ to equal work time
Very fit	>16 minutes	4–5 seconds	4–6	½ to equal work time
Maximal intervals				
Beginner	4–6 minutes	6–60 seconds	variable	variable
Quite fit	6–10 minutes	6–90 seconds	variable	variable
Very fit	>10 minutes	6–120 seconds	variable	variable

ENDURANCE TRAINING CATEGORIES IN RELATION TO EXERCISE INTENSITY AND DURATION

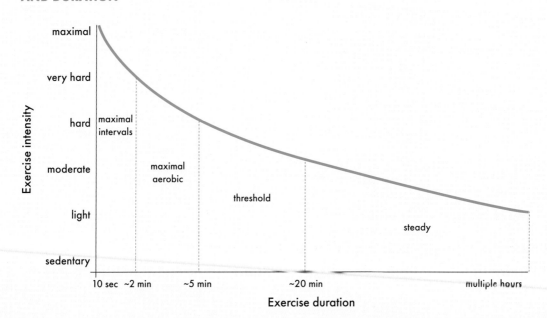

Strength and power training

Strength training is the other principal form of training utilised for its performance, appearance and health benefits. It is classically associated with getting bigger, stronger, faster and more powerful and therefore key to improving sports performance. In contrast, its value to health and general fitness is frequently underestimated. Strength training promotes being lean, as muscle tissue has a high metabolic rate. Therefore, when you tone or create new muscle, you are burning more calories all the time, even when sleeping. Strength training is also great for our health as it reduces the natural deficits of ageing associated with strength and bone health, helping us to maintain an independent lifestyle, and it is effective in preventing common metabolic diseases, such as type-2 diabetes. Strength training is great for preventing injuries, as it enables muscles and joints to cope with greater levels of force, and can improve posture, flexibility and muscle activation patterns. Thankfully, the tide is turning, and it's great to see as many women as men in the weights room, with activities such as CrossFit becoming increasingly popular, and both old and young reaping the benefits of strength training.

The amount and speed of the force involved in a strength exercise has different effects on the muscles, nerves and hormonal systems that dictate our training adaptations. Colour-Fit strength training categorises training based on these different training effects, and it thereby simplifies choosing the optimal strength training methods to achieve your goals.

Categories of Colour-Fit strength training

Strength Endurance generally involves lighter weights or bodyweight exercises performed for higher repetitions (more than 12), which improves our *endurance*/ability to perform more reps. Strength endurance makes our joint structures more robust and causes modest improvements in muscle size and strength. It is therefore a good starting point for anyone new to strength training and forms a base from which to progress to more intensive training. The use of higher reps means that there are potential fitness, health and weight management benefits, particularly if we perform exercises in a circuit fashion with little rest, as is done in many exercise classes.

Strength Size training aims to increase the *size* of the working muscles. This is the typical reason that most of us do strength training: to look athletic and to have toned muscles. Muscle size also has a large effect on the strength capacity and is therefore popular in performance-based training. Muscle growth is stimulated by both the force and the metabolite build-up that a muscle is exposed to. Therefore, strength size training aims to elicit both these stimuli by using exercises that involve high forces but can be performed a sufficient number of times to cause metabolic build up. The optimal load for this is about 6–12 repetitions performed to fatigue. Strength Size training often uses clever tweaks to training structures to maximise the stimuli for muscle growth, some of which are discussed in the Muscle Growth training plan.

Strength Max training aims to make us as strong as possible for a given movement. It involves high forces so movements can only be performed for a low number of repetitions (1–5) which lead to neural adaptions that allow us to create more force. The low reps and limited build-up of metabolites means that we get stronger without increasing muscle size too much. This allows us to be strong but as light as possible, which is key in most fitness and sport activities, because we must move our bodyweight around against gravity. A by-product of increased maximum strength is enhanced endurance, because we are able to use a lower percentage of our strength for a given action, so we become more efficient (in other words, it is easier). To ensure high force exposure, Strength Max training utilises multiple sets with long rests between sets so that we can train with maximum intensity throughout.

Power is a product of force multiplied by velocity, and therefore involves either lower load exercises where we can move quickly, referred to as **Speed Strength** (for example jumps, throws, sprints), or move heavier weights at speed, referred to as **Strength Speed** (for example Olympic lifts). Most sporting actions, such as throws, sprints and jumps involve developing force in extremely short time frames (less than 0.2 seconds). Only strength power training is effective at improving strength and/or velocity capability in such a short time, and it is therefore key to sports with high power movements. High power also means high energy expenditure, so this type of training is increasingly used for fitness and weight management, in cross-training and Tabata-like circuits.

BENEFITS AND STRUCTURE OUTLINE FOR THE STRENGTH TRAINING METHODS

max = maximum weight for 1 rep (see page 201 for other abbreviations)

Method	Benefits	Intensity/% max	Reps	Sets	Rest
Strength endurance	• Increase muscular endurance • Robust joints and muscles • Potential high calorie burn • CV health effects	• Light-to-moderate • <70% max	>12	1–5	0–60 seconds
Strength size	• Increase muscle size and strength • Increase resting metabolic rate	• Heavy • 70–85% max	6–12	2–5	30 seconds–3 minutes
Strength max	• Increase strength • Secondary effects on power and endurance • Some gain in muscle size	• Very heavy • >80% max	1–5	3–5	3–4 minutes
Speed strength	• Increase power and speed • Potential high calorie burn	• Bodyweight 50% max	5–10	3–6	3–4 minutes
Strength speed	• Increase power and speed • Potential high calorie burn	• Heavy >80% max	1–5	3–6	3–4 minutes

Colour-Fit Training Principles

Now that you know all about the different Colour-Fit training methods, you need to know how to best use them to achieve your goals. Methods are many, but principles are few, so if you grasp the principles below, it will help you to select the optimum training methods throughout your varied health and fitness journey.

You've got to push, and then push a bit more

We've known about the fundamental principles of training since ancient Greek times: overload and progression. The essence of training is to overload the body so that it is taken out of its comfort zone. The body does not like to be stressed, so it makes changes in order that the stress is no longer stressful – in other words we get fitter/stronger. Unfortunately, this means that you can't just sit in the sauna to get fitter, and you have to get comfortable with being uncomfortable. To get continually fitter, we must progressively make training harder so that it still represents a stress on the body. Furthermore, each progressively more intense training method serves as a building block on which you can better develop more intense fitness qualities. Therefore, it makes sense to progress overall training load gradually over time as you get fitter and progress from lower to higher intensity training methods. In addition to long-term fitness gains, this is a safe way to progressively load your muscles and joints so that you don't get injured.

If you are just starting out on your fitness journey, lower intensity methods will be challenging enough for you, and training two to four times per week will result in good fitness gains. As you get fitter, you can perform more intense and longer training sessions, and you will recover faster so you can exercise more frequently.

Train specifically for your goals – but not too much!

Specificity is another key training principle. We adapt specifically to the stress placed upon the body. Therefore, we should principally train specific movements and physiological systems that suit our goals. Colour-Fit Training is designed to help you select the best training methods intuitively, but the table on the following page also helps you to choose the principal training methods to achieve common training goals.

Goal	Endurance method	Strength method
Lose fat	Steady (calories) and maximal intervals (metabolism)	Strength endurance (calorie burn)
Muscle growth	n/a	Strength size
Health	Steady (calories) and maximal intervals (metabolism)	Strength endurance (calorie burn) and size (metabolism)
Long events (e.g. marathon)	Steady	Strength max (economy)
Medium event (10km run)	Threshold and maximal aerobic	Strength max (economy)
Short events (e.g. 100m row)	Maximal intervals	Power and strength max
Prolonged sport (e.g. football, hockey)	All endurance methods	Strength max and power

Specificity also relates to using movements similar to those used in our goal activity, so we train appropriate neuromuscular pathways, and develop technical and tactical proficiency at the same time. Therefore, rowers should mainly row, tennis players play tennis, and so on. Performance strength training should predominantly use exercises with similar movements and muscles to those performed in your chosen sport. The use of free weights (for example dumbbells, barbells, cables, kettlebells, medicine balls) rather than fixed machines is a good way to achieve this. The table below lists some of the key free-weight strength exercises with a link to video demonstrations.

Body section	Strength/power exercises	Video link
Leg strength	Deadlift, squat, 1-leg squat, step-up, lunge, rear-foot elevated squat	
Leg posterior strength	Romanian dead lifts, Nordics, glut thrusts	
Leg power	Jumps/hops, squat jump, step-up jumps, Olympic lifts	
Upper-body push	Bench, push-up, cable push, shoulder press, dips, throws	
Upper-body pull	Row, cable pull, pull-ups, upright row	
Core	Bridges/planks, cable woodchop and rotations, deadbugs, Norwegian groins, palloffs	

Despite the law of specificity, a certain level of mixing training methods, rather than always using the same method, has been shown to produce superior results. The body responds more to varied stimuli because it is easier to adapt to just one type of training, so it no longer stresses the body. Furthermore, many of the different training methodologies interact – for example muscle size affects maximum strength – and different fitness qualities are often needed at different stages of a race or match (for example a sprint finish in a marathon; a scrum versus a sprint for a try).

Rest up for results

It sounds strange, but if we want to get fitter, rest is as important as training! It is during rest periods that our bodies use energy to restore and enhance the numerous bodily systems that are stressed during training. We also need time to recover from fatigue so that we can train optimally again and reduce the risk of injury. Training load and intensity are the principal determinants for required recovery times. Lower intensity methods, such as Steady Endurance and Strength Endurance, only need about a day to recover from unless you have performed a really challenging session. Therefore, you can generally perform lower intensity methods more frequently and closer to important performance events. Higher intensity methods and hard sessions generally need about two days before you can effectively recover for further high-intensity training or competition, unless the duration of training is relatively short. A person with greater training experience will recover quicker than a novice. We all know the dreaded aches and pains when we haven't trained for a while. Also, younger people generally recover quicker than us older folks. Finally, we tend to recover more quickly from unweighted forms of training, such as swimming and cycling, than loaded methods such as running, especially if it involves intense actions such as a rapid change of direction and collisions, as are common in sports such as rugby and ice hockey.

When you are approaching an important event (for example a race or match day) that you have been training towards for some time, you would typically enter what is known as a 'taper' – a period during which the amount of overall training is reduced – so that you reach the big day as fresh and as fit as possible. Generally, the more demanding the training regime and the event, the longer the taper period required, due to the greater stresses the body has gone through. For example, a typical marathon training programme would require a 2-week taper because of the extensive training required and the toll of the final preparation run, whereas a 5km run would only require a 1–3-day taper.

These days there are endless methods and gadgets that aim to hasten recovery times so that we can train again sooner or be fresher for competition. Good nutrition and sleep will always be the foundations of recovery. Sleep for optimal recovery varies between people, but generally you should aim for 7–9 hours and to be asleep by 11pm to maximise deep sleep. The upcoming nutrition plans provide lots of nutritional tips for maximising recovery.

PART 3
COLOUR-FIT PLANS

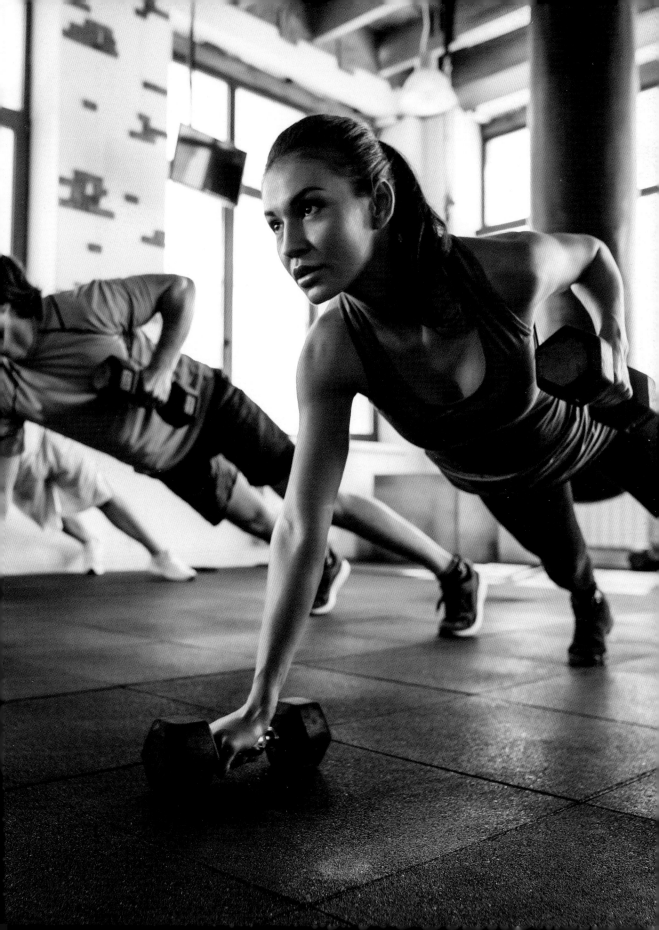

Colour-Fit Plans bring the Cook and Training components of the book together by providing training and meal plans to help you achieve a range of goals. My team and I have expertly designed a range of fitness and sport training plans that include running, cycling, triathlon and skill-based sports such as football and rugby. In addition, you'll find plans focusing on the body-shape goals of becoming lean/fat loss and gaining muscle, plus a health-boosting plan.

Navigating the plans

The training programmes cater for beginners, right through to elite athletes, so they will result in optimal fitness and performance gains no matter what your level. All our programmes are based on science-backed evidence and countless success stories of personal and sporting glory. The complementary meal plans are meticulously designed to achieve the desired goals and support optimum training and performance, while maximising health, taste and practicality. Here are some important elements we've included in the plans to help you navigate them more easily.

Training Load Gauges

Within the plans, you'll find the Colour-Fit Training Load Gauges, which use colours and icons to provide quick, intuitive information about training as follows:

1 The type of training We use icons to represent the type of training, and colours to reflect the different types of endurance training: lower intensity training has a cooler colour while more intense training has hotter colours (so blue for lower intensity through to dark red for high intensity). For some training methods, the training intensity is very changeable (for example, strength, CrossFit, circuits, spinning, skill-sport training), therefore for these we use a grey colour to represent a generic training load.

TRAINING LOAD/INTENSITY

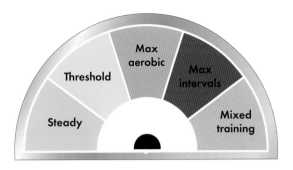

TRAINING TYPE ICONS

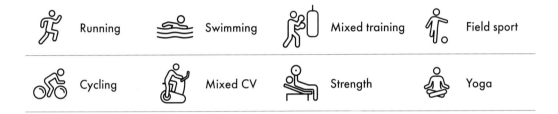

Running	Swimming	Mixed training	Field sport
Cycling	Mixed CV	Strength	Yoga

2 How hard the training will be (the training load) Assessing training load can be complex. It is essentially training duration multiplied by training intensity but requires that intensity is considered on an exponential scale, and the mode of training also needs to be considered. Training gauges simplify training load, with a fuller gauge indicating a harder training session and vice-versa. The fullness of each colour also represents the proportional load from each training type. Where Training Load Gauges are not appropriate, we give a description of approximate training load.

Training load term	Description
Very easy	Light activity for moderate time, no fatigue
Easy	Low-to-moderate intensity or short-duration session, low fatigue
Moderate	Challenging session, some fatigue
Hard	Intense or prolonged exercise, high fatigue
Very hard	Exhausted, rest required

Here are some examples of Colour-Fit Training Load gauges.

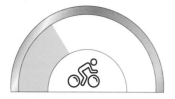

Bike – steady training with
an **easy** training load

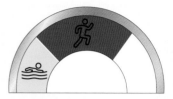

Swim – threshold for an **easy** load
Run – max intervals
with a moderate-hard load

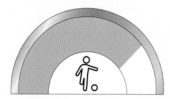

Football – max aerobic training
with a **moderate-hard** training load

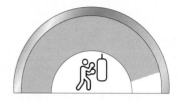

Circuit – mixed training with
a **very hard** training load

I provide rationales for each plan so that you can understand the principles they are based on and adapt them to suit your tastes and lifestyle. Each plan is designed as a guide and not a precise prescriptive tool. Each of us will have individual requirements and preferences and we need to take account of those to make the plans work for us. When following the training plans, if aches and pains start to increase or your mood and sleep deteriorate, ease off the overall volume for a while and perhaps start with a lower training load.

For the meal plans I have deliberately provided a wide variety of meals to inspire you and to give several suitable examples, but in reality few of us have this much variety in our diet, so don't worry about repeating the same meals a few times throughout the week. Most of the meals suggested are for recipes in this book, but you'll also find the occasional simple suggestion such as crackers and cottage cheese or steak. I hope you don't feel you need a recipe for those! Meal plans do not contain drinks, small snacks or supplements that would contribute to the overall calorie load, and therefore they are deliberately designed to be a bit light on normal calorie recommendations. It is difficult to give advice on exact portion size/servings because everyone has different body sizes, genetics, activity levels and goals. In general, if you eat the suggested foods conscientiously to satisfy your hunger, while taking time to enjoy your food, your caloric intake should be roughly appropriate. Again, monitoring things like your health, body shape and energy levels and adjusting accordingly is important.

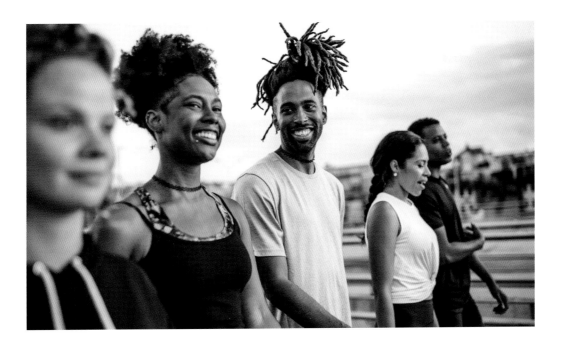

Many experts suggest tracking macros – the amount of carbs, proteins and fats we consume – to individualise your diet and meet your nutritional goals. While it can be useful, macro-tracking is difficult and can detract from food enjoyment. Remember, Colour-Fit is about enjoying food and being in the right ball park, most of the time. However, the more demanding your performance or body-shape goal, the more some short-term macro tracking may help to ensure your training and dietary needs are met. The table below gives my recommendations for macros following three main principles:

1. With increasing activity demands, increase your carb intake, and slightly increase protein and fat.
2. For weight loss, increase your protein and reduce fat and carbs.
3. For muscle growth, increase your carbs and protein, and slightly increase fat.

Training/ Activity	Sedentary	Moderate– hard	Hard– extreme	Fuel for competition	Weight loss	Muscle growth
Carbs (g/kg)	2–4	3–6	5–10	5–8	1.5–5 *	4–8 *
Protein (g/kg)	1–1.6	1.5–2	2–2.5	1–1.6	2–3	1.6–3
Fats (g/kg)	0.5–1	0.8–1.2	1–2.5	0.5–0.8	0.5–0.8	1–1.5

* weight loss and muscle growth carb recommendations are training dependent
g/kg represent grams per kilogram of body weight

Now is the time to take action and achieve your goals, so let's dive into the plans.

Health Plan

Good health is something that many of us take for granted until we fall into ill-health. But heed my words: the greatest investment you can make in life *right now*, is in your health. Adopting the principles in this plan will help you achieve enhanced mood, appearance, mobility, immunity, brain function, libido and longevity – the list goes on. A healthy life equals a happy life, and it certainly doesn't have to be boring – I can party with the best of them!

To construct the health plan, I teamed up with renowned well-being company Hero Wellbeing. They provide a holistic model of physical, social, mental and nutritional support through their Navigator app, on-site services and training clubs, and I'm very proud that Colour-Fit is the foundation of their nutritional provision.

Training plan: health

There are an abundance of training methods that you can use to optimise your health. Advice from the World Health Organization (WHO) is that you perform any exercise for about 30 minutes most days. This can be as simple as walking to work or gardening. Any of the training methods discussed in this book could be considered healthy as they encourage calorie burning, improved muscle function and boost cardiovascular, metabolic, hormonal and mental health. The key to health is sustainability, so find something you enjoy. My top tips for enjoyment are to exercise with friends, exercise in beautiful surroundings (where possible) and combine exercise with something else you enjoy, such as listening to music/podcasts, watching a programme or reading a book. Pretty much any activity will be beneficial to your physical and mental health: dancing, walking in Mother Nature, trampolining with the kids, exercise classes with a friend, cleaning the house (maybe not the last one); however, the training methods utilised in the plan below have secondary benefits for our health beyond general fitness. The plan is suitable for anyone and is designed to fit in with our busy lifestyles.

The 'fast' track to health

Endurance training, in particular steady training, has been shown to provide several health benefits, such as reduced blood pressure, healthier heart and arteries and better metabolic health. An issue can be that steady training requires relatively long training times. However, a solution when time is tight is to exercise in a fasted state (an extended period where you do not take on calories), such as in the morning before breakfast. Fasted endurance training has been shown to produce slightly greater benefits relating to fitness, metabolic health and longevity, when compared to training in a fed state, so you can get results in a shorter time frame. Fasted training should not be highly exertive for your level of fitness, as the lower levels of available energy increase the risk of fatigue and injury. When you want to push levels of intensity and exertion a bit further, it is better to be fuelled for the session. Furthermore, by far the most important factor for health is that you exercise, rather than be in a fasted state, so if you haven't got the time or energy in the morning, simply exercise later in the day. Extensive steady training will provide cardiovascular benefits, such as a more elastic heart and greater blood volume, resulting in reduced blood pressure. If you are feeling brave, you could try open-water swimming for your aerobic exercise, as it has recently been associated with protective effects for the brain against dementia.

The lunch-break blast

In our busy lifestyles, it can be hard to fit in exercise; however, intense maximal intervals are very time efficient and effective for boosting fitness and metabolism. Exercising for just 4 minutes using Tabata intervals (20 seconds exercise, 10 seconds rest) has been shown to be as effective as 30 minutes steady exercise for improvements in fitness, weight loss and blood-health markers, so get your shorts ready for your lunch break.

Strengthen your health

Many people do not associate strength training with health benefits, but this is far from the case. Natural deficits caused by ageing relate to muscle strength, bone density and circulating levels of hormones that are boosted by strength training. Metabolic diseases, such as type-2 diabetes, represent one of the largest health concerns in the world. Strength training provides a key strategy against these diseases by stimulating a range of muscles to use carbohydrates effectively; inefficient use of carbohydrates by the body is a common issue in metabolic diseases and leads to a catalogue of health issues. As this plan is for everyone, the strength training uses mainly body weight exercises that can be done with minimal equipment at home (only a mini-band is required) and is designed to improve our ability to perform daily functions. The plan predominantly uses strength-endurance exercises performed in a circuit fashion, so you achieve strength and cardiovascular benefits simultaneously. (Scan the QR codes for video demonstrations of the circuits.)

Stretch your mental well-being

The benefits of yoga have been recognised for centuries. Yoga improves mobility, strength and posture, encourages good breathing patterns, and lowers stress hormones, such as cortisol, which wreak havoc in our bodies due to our modern busy lives. The plan has two yoga sessions provided by the brilliant Gavin DeMarines from Hero Training Clubs, with video links to the sessions.

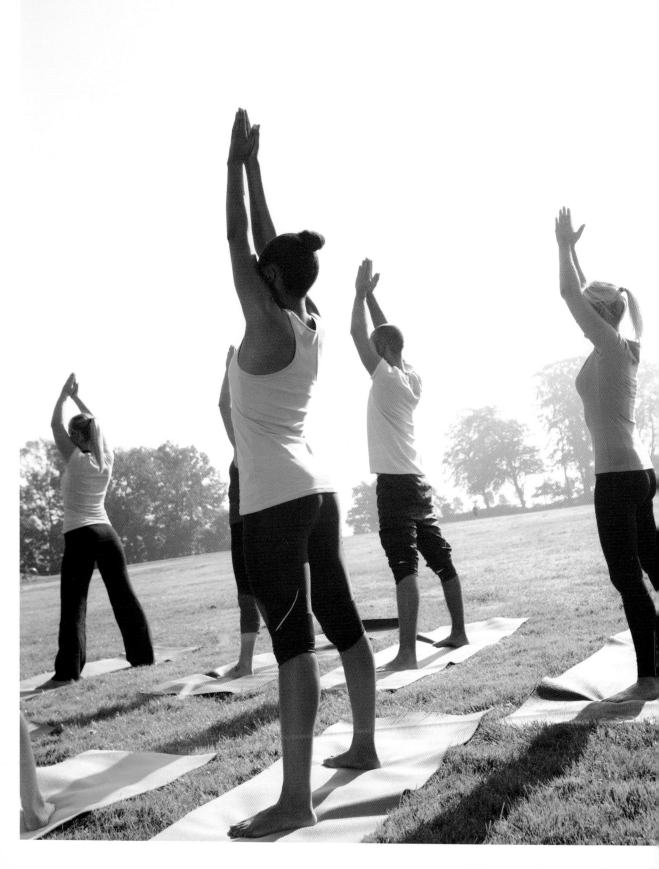

HEALTH SCHEDULE

Day	Training Load Gauge	Training	QR code
Monday		**Yoga session 1**	
Tuesday		**Strength endurance circuit 1:** 3–4 rounds. 10 reps of each exercise: burpees, speed squats, T-rotation push-ups, ice skaters, mountain climbers, lawn mower squat, bear kick-throughs	
Wednesday		**Tabata maximal intervals:** 8–12 × 20 seconds maximal effort, 10 seconds rest any exercise; e.g. run, bike/spin, row, CV machine	n/a
Thursday		**Yoga session 2**	
Friday		**Strength endurance circuit 2:** 3–4 rounds. 10 reps of each exercise: high knees, push-ups, lunge squat, leg drops, cook bridge. Mini-band circuit: side walks, kick-backs, band squat, band bridge, deadbugs	
Saturday		**Pre-breakfast extensive steady:** 30–60 minutes steady endurance exercise; e.g. run, bike/spin, swim, row, CV machine	n/a
Sunday		Rest	n/a

Training bar key: steady threshold  max aerobic max intervals mixed training

Meal plan: health

Unsurprisingly, the focus of the health meal plan is to provide lots of meals that are high in Health and have high health scores. As nutrition is so critical to our health, I expand on some more generic information for healthy nutrition after the plan.

	Monday	Tuesday	Wednesday
	Training Yoga **Training load** Easy **Rationale** Health	**Training** Circuit **Training load** Moderate **Rationale** Balanced to support exercise, health and recovery	**Training** Tabata **Training load** Moderate **Rationale** Health bias; Fuel around Tabata
Breakfast	Green Shakshuka (page 55)	Poached Eggs in Tomato (page 49)	Smoked Salmon and Guacamole Toast (page 44)
Morning snack	No snack	No snack	No snack
Lunch	Beetroot and Apple Salad with Smoked Tofu (page 67)	Mediterranean Wraps (page 76)	Spanish Tomato Salad (page 69)
Afternoon snack	Apple	Almond and Ginger Smoothie (page 189)	Lettuce and Tuna Boats (page 156)
Dinner	Hake with Sautéed Vegetables (page 100)	Almond-Breaded Chicken Strips and Cabbage Salad (pages 72 and 136)	Minute Steak with Roast Peppered and Avocado Salad (page 129)
Evening snack	No snack	No snack	No snack

Thursday	Friday	Saturday	Sunday
Training Yoga **Training load** Easy **Rationale** Health bias as calorie demands are low	**Training** Circuit **Training load** Moderate **Rationale** Balanced to support exercise, health and recovery	**Training** Fasted steady **Training load** Moderate–easy **Rationale** Balanced to support exercise, health and recovery	**Training** Rest **Training load** n/a **Rationale** Health and Lean Muscle bias as calorie demands are low
Courgette Pancakes (page 52)	Mango and Banana Parfait (page 30)	Healthy English Breakfast (page 51)	Avocado Baked Eggs (page 47)
No snack	No snack	No snack	No snack
Prawn and Asparagus Stir-Fry (page 71)	Ham, Avocado and Egg Wrap (page 77)	Asian-Style Super Salad (page 64)	Broccoli and Mint Soup (page 61)
Hummus and chopped pepper	Courgette and Turkey Rolls (page 157)	Berries and Greek yogurt	Joint Jellies (page 160)
Thai Fishcakes and Sweet-and-Sour Crispy Asian Sprouts (pages 106 and 153)	Autumn Chicken and Veggie Bake (page 109)	Slow-Cooker Butternut Squash and Lentil Curry (page 93)	Lemon Sea Bass and Asparagus Bake (page 105)
No snack	No snack	No snack	No snack

Some guiding principles

'Nutrition is healthcare, whilst medicine is sick care' is a quote that has stuck with me and exemplifies how critical nutrition is to our health. As such, I felt it best to expand on some nutritional health information below.

Eat as Mother Nature intended

A simple rule for healthy eating is to mainly eat foods as they are found in nature. We evolved over millions of years eating foods in their natural state that we could forage, hunt or grow. With natural foods, it is not just the individual nutrients within them that are important for our health but how they combine and are contained within the food. The alteration of natural food, known as processing, such as milling, pasteurisation and canning, has brought us huge benefits in terms of food availability and convenience. However, the prevalence of modern food manufacturing practices has led to a sharp rise in the consumption of *ultra*-processed foods, which have added ingredients that are bad for our health, such as sugar, hydrogenated fats/oils, salt, artificial flavourings and preservatives, and a lack of healthy elements such as fibre. The purpose of ultra-processing is typically to make foods cheaper, more stable and more palatable, and therefore highly desirable and convenient. It is this high-level processing of foods that is damaging to our health, with a worrying statistic that about 70 per cent of the foods in the typical Western diet are ultra-processed. Check food labels, and if a food contains lots of ingredients that you do not recognise, it's probably not a healthy choice. Most healthy foods don't need a nutrition label because you are buying them in their natural form.

Numerous studies have shown that diets rich in wholefoods, such as vegetables, fruit, beans, lentils, wholegrains, nuts and seeds are associated with healthier lives. These plant foods contain a variety of vitamins, minerals, fibre and phytonutrients, which protect plants from damage and disease and have a similar effect for us when we consume them. Try to eat a wide range of different coloured plant foods to provide the best range of nutrients. In addition to making food taste great, herbs and spices are rich in phytonutrients, so the regular use of these is highly recommended for our health as well as our taste buds.

Improving health by increasing vegetable intake has always been my main battleground when working with athletes. However, it is always worth the effort – learning how delicious vegetables can be with the use of herbs and spices, and including them in simple stir-fry, casserole and curry dishes, has always resulted improved performance, waistlines and overall well-being.

Be canny with your carbs

Carbs are a divisive subject and their role in the body is often misunderstood. When we eat carbs they are broken down into glucose and absorbed by the blood to be transported to where they can be used directly for energy or stored. The rise in blood glucose after eating carbs causes the release of insulin, which promotes the storage of glucose in our muscles and liver, thereby lowering blood glucose, plus the storage of fats and protein. How quickly a food raises our blood glucose is known as glycaemic index – a high glycaemic index food would raise it quickly, causing a more prominent insulin response and increased storage. Glycaemic load is the amount of carbs in a serving and more accurately reflects the effect of a food on blood glucose concentration.

Issues arise if we are inactive and frequently eat high-glycaemic foods because our storage system becomes full. Blood glucose therefore remains elevated and the excess has to be converted to fat, both of which are damaging to our health. Also, because insulin remains elevated, we begin to produce less and become desensitised to it, creating a vicious spiral where we cannot deal with carb foods effectively, and develop type-2 diabetes. It is estimated that approximately 50 per cent of the US population now has diabetes or prediabetes, with Europe following closely behind.

Carbs that are made of refined grains, such as white breads, pasta, cereals and pastries have a high glycaemic index. Carb foods that contain fibre have a lower glycaemic index, such as wholemeal versions of the breads and pastas, wholegrains such as quinoa, brown rice, barley, oats and buckwheat, and vegetables. These foods are absorbed by the digestive system more slowly, thereby sustaining our energy, staving off hunger for longer, and helping to control our blood glucose.

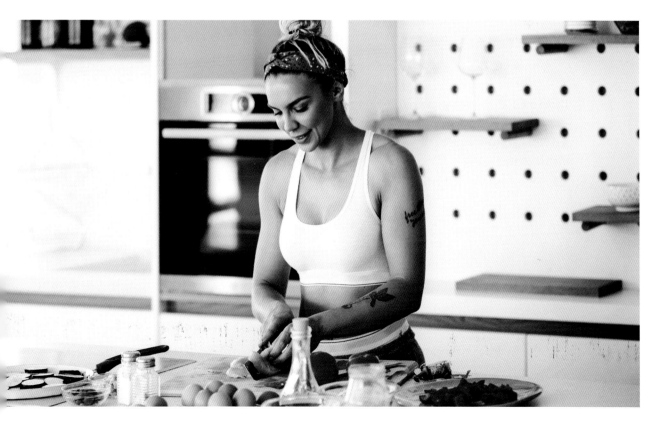

Foods high in sugars also have a high glycaemic index. Of course, sugar exists naturally in things such as fruit and dairy, but consuming these is generally fine as we digest these more slowly (because fibre and protein slow the absorption of sugar). Free sugar – manufactured sugar that is added to foods – is absorbed into our blood very quickly. Free sugar is also highly palatable and can be packed together tightly, making foods very calorie dense and easy to overeat, leading to weight gain, in addition to causing tooth decay. It goes without saying that we should therefore moderate sugary foods and drinks, such as confectionery, cakes, cereals and sodas. Check your food labels and look out for ingredients ending in 'ose' and syrups. Sweeteners can sometimes be used as a substitute, but they are not without their issues. Sweet spices such as cinnamon and cardamom can be a good alternative and are beneficial for our health.

Don't be flummoxed by fats

Fats are a topic of much debate and confusion, to the extent that the advice – like many nutritional topics – seems to be ever-changing. One thing is widely accepted, however: despite being demonised because of their association with *being* fat and chronic diseases, fats – or more precisely fatty acids – play an essential role in a healthy diet, being critical to cell structure and signalling, brain function, energy provision, hormone production, immune function and many more important tasks.

There are numerous different types of fats but they are most commonly divided into saturated fats, found in animal-based foods such as meat and dairy (and often high in confectionery such as biscuits and chocolate); monounsaturated fats, found in olive oil, rapeseed oil, avocado and some nuts; polyunsaturated fats, which is a wide group covering everything from the fats in oily fish to those in flaxseed; and partially hydrogenated fats (often called trans fats), a type of fat used in processed foods.

Current UK recommendations are that total fat should make up less than 35 per cent of our total calorie intake per day, less than 11 per cent of that should come from saturated fat, and we should minimise our intake of trans fat. What do I take from that basic message? Yes, limit your intake of saturated fat as per the guidelines, as an excess over time is associated with cardiovascular risks and inflammation, but, when you do eat it, opt for quality sources like grass-fed meat and organic dairy, as they will provide a lot of other beneficial nutrients. When it comes to unsaturated fats think olive oil, avocado, nuts and seeds but, most particularly, include those fatty fish such as salmon, mackerel and trout which contain a particularly important type of fatty acid, omega-3. And whereas cooking oils such as olive and rapeseed contain unsaturated fats and are recommended (notwithstanding that proviso to limit total fat intake), other vegetable oils, such as sunflower oil, contain less healthy fats. Partially hydrogenated fats should be avoided. They were originally designed as an industrial lubricant, and unsurprisingly are not processed well by the body. They are used in food processing to increase shelf life and add texture, so limit foods like bars, confectionery and ultra-processed foods.

Meat your health needs

Meat can be a controversial topic where health and the environment are concerned. Natural meat contains a range of nutrients, especially minerals, and organ meats are considered some of the most nutrient-dense foods we can eat. However, diets in developed countries typically contain sufficient protein and recommendations are generally to reduce the amount of meat we eat, though of course that depends on how much you eat in the first place. Protein is certainly key in any healthy diet as it forms the building blocks for all our cells and we rely on the dietary protein to obtain essential amino acids, which perform important structural and chemical processes in the body. Meat is a well absorbed protein that contains all the essential amino acids.

If you abstain from meat, you can get sufficient protein by consuming a variety of beans, wholegrains, legumes, soya and mycoprotein products – plus dairy and egg if you are vegetarian – but it requires careful thought and planning.

Processed meats, such as sausages and bacon, should be considered differently and consumed only in moderation because they are high in saturated fat, but also preservatives such as nitrites that are thought to be a cancer risk.

Hydrate for health

Our bodies are 45–75 per cent water, so it's not surprising that hydration is important to our health. Fortunately, we are well attuned to our water needs, so simply paying attention to our thirst and hydration levels should be adequate for most of us. Monitoring your urine colour is a good back-up method: if it's a strong yellow, and particularly if it's dark and smelly, drink more water. When exercising, we lose more fluids through sweat, especially in hot and humid conditions, and we should therefore aim to drink more and to potentially use electrolytes (in pre-made sport drinks or add an electrolyte tablet) to help retain fluids and replace sodium lost in sweat.

Water, with or without a sugar-free flavouring, should be our main drink choice. Green tea, tea and coffee contain healthy phytonutrients, and moderate levels of caffeine are good for us, so up to three to five cups a day is fine; however, limit caffeine intake if you find it makes you jittery, and avoid it later in the day so that your sleep is not disturbed. Moderate your intake of sugary beverages, such as sodas, energy drinks and fruit concentrates, because they are calorie dense and bad for our teeth. Alcohol should ideally be consumed in moderation, too, as it is fairly calorie dense; furthermore, it causes inflammation and an excess damages the liver. Red wine does contain some healthy phytonutrients, so it can be consumed in moderation, note *moderation*, as part of a healthy diet.

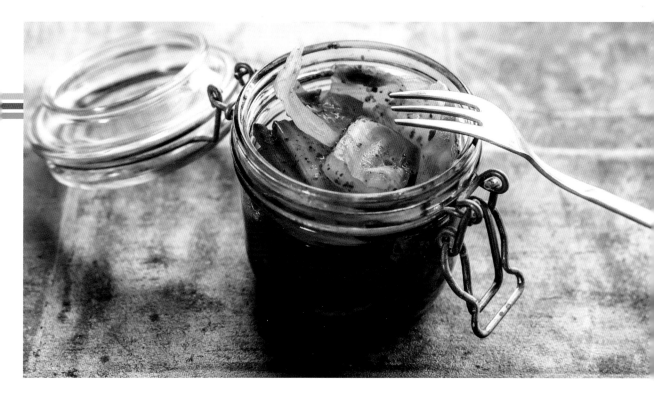

Follow your gut

Gut health is an exciting new frontier in nutritional science. Our guts house trillions of microbes that form about two-thirds of our immune cells. These microbes produce important nutrients and signal molecules, which act on the brain and hormonal systems, and as such affect our immunity, mood, energy and body composition. It's complex stuff, but thankfully the practical recommendations are pretty simple and familiar: eat a range of different-coloured vegetables, fruit and wholegrains, which provide a variety of fibres to feed our good gut bacteria; avoid too much sugar and processed foods because these promote bad bacteria in the gut (as well as creating other problems, as we saw earlier). If you have gut issues, consuming probiotic foods that contain good gut bacteria, such as yogurts and fermented foods (kimchi and sauerkraut), might help.

Be inclusive, not exclusive

In modern food-health marketing, we see the term 'free from' a lot, be it gluten from grains or lactose from diary – so much so that you would think it must be essential to exclude these to have a healthy diet. You might have also heard of things such as oxalates, phytates and lectins found in fruits, vegetables and pulses, which some proponents of nutrition say we should avoid; however, within normal consumption, these food groups are good for us. Food intolerances are rare and avoiding food groups unnecessarily could lead to you missing out on important nutrients – as well reducing your enjoyment of food. If you have an intolerance or allergy, you would have fairly persistent symptoms, such as stomach issues, rashes and inflammation, and should therefore seek the advice of a doctor or dietician.

Fat-Loss/Lean Plan

This fat-loss plan will help you to shed some pounds and improve your general fitness so that you look and feel great. Virtually all of us have started a diet or training regime with the aim of losing weight – be it for a holiday, a special occasion or to improve our health. We have an innate biological drive to be as attractive as possible to lure a mate, and that's without the ever-increasing pressures of modern society requiring us to look slim and athletic. More importantly, being overweight is now the primary cause of early mortality in developed countries with 30–50 per cent of people clinically obese. Rather than losing weight, I prefer to talk about losing fat, because it is excess *fat* that leads to ill-health and not all weight is the same – we want to keep muscle weight to maintain metabolism, and many diets obtain weight loss via body water reduction, which is only short term.

Essentially, fat loss and gain are a game of calorie balance: calories in from food and drink versus calories out from bodily functions and physical activity. If we burn more calories than we consume, then we lose weight, and vice versa. The phrase often used is 'eat less, move more', but I prefer 'eat smart, move smart', as there are several intricacies to losing fat effectively in the long term, which we will explore.

The fat-loss plan is suitable for a beginner right through to a fitness enthusiast, but a very fit person may want something more challenging. If this is you, simply add some more training sessions throughout the week.

Training plan: fat loss/lean

The aim of the training plan is to increase the amount of calories we burn, targeting calories from fat, in a time-efficient manner that suits our busy lifestyles. It involves circuits that require some standard equipment found in any gym or that you could purchase for use at home: dumbbells, barbells and a box/raised surface. Videos of the circuit exercises can be viewed via the QR codes. Any variety of high-intensity training classes, such as spin, HIIT or Tabata, could be swapped for the circuits, if you like.

Slow and steady wins the race

When training at a steady pace, we can keep going for long periods and thereby burn lots of calories. Lower intensity exercise also means a greater percentage of energy is supplied from fat because higher intensities require energy production rates beyond what fat can support, relying on the more rapid energy production of carbohydrates. Therefore, the plan uses predominantly Steady Endurance training. To maximise fat burning and time efficiency, two steady sessions are recommended in a fasted state pre-breakfast. Lower carbohydrate stores and insulin levels upon waking, as a result of going without food for a sustained period while we sleep, boosts our ability to utilise fat for energy if we exercise before breakfast. If you haven't got time in the morning, actually performing the exercise is by far the critical aspect, so exercise at some point later in the day; plus you might have time for a longer session to burn more calories. The final steady session is performed post-fueling so we are able to perform a long duration session for extra calorie burning, and it's performed on the weekend when most of us have more spare time. For strength training we predominantly use Strength Endurance, because the lower intensity means that we can perform higher reps in a circuit fashion using sequentially different parts of the body, with minimal rest, which increases the contribution of the aerobic system and thereby fat breakdown for energy.

Go hard to go home early and boost metabolism

We all have busy lifestyles, so maximising time efficiency is key to long-term success. Although we cannot sustain high-intensity methods for extensive periods, they can burn a large number of calories in a short time. High-intensity training allows us to burn more calories throughout the day by boosting our metabolism and making us less lethargic compared to longer training sessions. The circuits mix in higher intensity endurance training in the Max Aerobic and Max Intervals range. This method of combining strength and high intensity endurance is seen in many modern forms of training like CrossFit and HIIT circuits. The strength exercises are great for negating the losses in muscle mass that normally happen during periods of a negative calorie balance, and therefore helps to keep metabolism high.

Be active

Although there are optimum forms of exercise to lose fat, please bear in mind that any activity burns calories, so any form of exercise – doing chores, taking the stairs, walking to work, and so on – can help with weight maintenance.

FAT-LOSS/LEAN SCHEDULE

Day	Training Load Gauge	Training	QR code
Monday		**Pre-breakfast – extensive steady:** 30–60 minutes, e.g. run, bike/spin, swim, row or mixed CV	n/a
Tuesday (evening)		**Fat loss circuit 1 (perform full circuit as quickly as possible):** • *Box circuit* 2 sets of 10 reps: box jump, feet elevated push-up, 1-leg elevated squat, mountain climbers, step-ups, dips, RFES, pike handstand press or push-up • *Run/treadmill/run-on-spot* 5 sets of 30 seconds fast, 30 seconds rest/slow • *Barbell circuit* 5–20kg bar. 2 sets of 10 reps: back squat, shoulder press, front squat, bent row, thruster, upright row, barbell push-up, roll-out • *Boxing bag/pads*, shadow box or skip: 5 × 1-minute rounds, 30 second rest	
Wednesday		Rest day	n/a
Thursday		**Pre-breakfast – extensive steady:** 30–60 minutes, e.g. run, bike/spin, swim, row or mixed CV	n/a
Friday (evening)		**Fat loss circuit 2 (perform full circuit as quickly as possible):** 2–3 sets of each line of exercises below in sequence before progressing to the next line: • 10 x step-up, push-up, inverted row • 10 × lunge squat, dips, pull-ups • Hold 5–12kg dumbbells: 10 x squat, upright row, shoulder press Finish with 1km run or row, or 5km bike	
Saturday		**Extensive steady** Aim for over 1 hour e.g. run/hike, bike/spin, swim, row, CV machines or mix of above	n/a
Sunday		Rest day	n/a

Training bar key: steady threshold max aerobic ⬤ max intervals ⬤ mixed training

Meal plan: fat loss/lean

	Monday	Tuesday	Wednesday
	Training Pre-breakfast, steady **Training load** Easy–moderate **Rationale** Health and Lean Muscle take priority; some Fuel post-am cardio	**Training** Evening, mixed circuit 1 **Training load** Hard **Rationale** Health and Lean Muscle take priority; some Fuel for pm circuit	**Training** Rest day **Training load** n/a **Rationale** Health and Lean Muscle take priority
Breakfast	Mocha Parfait (page 30)	Breakfast Burrito (page 39)	Poached Eggs in Tomato (page 49)
Lunch	Easy Tuna Salad (page 68)	Mediterranean Wrap (page 76)	Tuscan Bean Soup (page 62)
Afternoon snack	Lean Strawberry Smoothie (page 188)	Crackers and cottage cheese	Ham-wrapped asparagus
Dinner	Lemon Sea Bass and Asparagus Bake and Curried Cauli Rice (pages 105 and 137)	Creamy Chicken, Quinoa and Broccoli Bake (page 111)	Hake with Sautéed Vegetables (page 100)

When it comes to weight loss, training definitely helps, but nutrition is king, so it is critical to get your nutrition right. The main nutrition principles of the lean plan are that it has moderate calories and a high proportion of Lean Muscle and Health foods. Fuel is generally low but varies with the amount of training. You'll find some useful principles after the plan on pages 230-3).

Thursday	Friday	Saturday	Sunday
Training Pre-breakfast, steady **Training load** Easy–moderate **Rationale** Health and Lean Muscle take priority; some Fuel post-am cardio	**Training** Evening, mixed circuit 2 **Training load** Hard **Rationale** Health and Lean Muscle take priority; some fuel for pm circuit	**Training** Morning, steady (long) **Training load** Moderate–hard **Rationale** Balanced approach overall	**Training** n/a **Training load** Rest day **Rationale** Health and Lean Muscle take priority
Almond and Banana Pancakes (page 39)	Scrambled egg and spinach	Vanilla and Blueberry Overnight Oats (page 38)	Ful and Poached Egg (page 35)
Asian-Style Super-Salad (page 64)	Tortilla Pizza (page 73) and side salad	Mango and Pineapple Salad (page 65)	Prawn and Asparagus Stir-Fry (page 71)
Joint Jellies (page 160)	Berries and Greek yogurt	Courgette and Turkey Rolls (page 157)	Lettuce and Tuna Boats (page 156)
Smoked Haddock Kedgeree (page 101)	Turkey Burger with Feta and Spinach and Leeks, Peas and Quinoa (pages 118 and 145)	Sweet Potato Cottage Pie (page 124)	Minute Steak with Roasted Peppers and Avocado Salad (page 129)

Some guiding principles

Cut the calories

Exercise can help us create a negative calorie balance, but it takes a surprising amount of exercise to burn calories, plus when we train really hard our bodies can reduce our non-exercise calorie burning. It does this by reducing what's called non-exercise activity thermogenesis – by doing things like fidgeting less and being generally more lethargic. When we have a sustained large negative calorie balance the body also reduces our resting metabolic rate by taking energy away from things like sex hormones and bone formation in order to prioritise staying alive. Given all that, limiting the calories we consume is definitely the key route to fat loss.

The majority of the meals in the plan have a moderate-to-low calorie load, using mainly low-calorie-dense food, such as non-starchy vegetables (the main starchy vegetables are potatoes, parsnip, peas and butternut squash), salads and lean protein sources, such as lean meat and fish. Fat has over double the calories of carbs and proteins, therefore the plan limits the amount of unhealthy fats while allowing some essential healthy fats, such as those found in nuts, seeds, avocado and fish, that are key to our health (see page 222 for more on fats). You can also use reduced-fat dairy and dressings or sauces, cut away visible fat, use a spray for cooking oils and steam/roast/air-fry rather than fry. The plan limits sugary foods and drinks, in addition to foods that combine refined carbs and fat, such as baking products, confectionery and fast foods, as they are very calorie dense and palatable, so we tend to overeat them.

A calorie deficit of around 10–20 per cent over a sustained period has been found to be more effective long term than larger calorie deficits, as these cause excessive hunger and the protective drop in our metabolism outlined earlier. This deficit would produce a weight loss of around 0.5kg per week, although you are likely to lose less as time goes on. Assessing appropriate calorie intake is complex, even with elaborate testing, as it depends on several varying factors, such as genetics, weight, activity levels, sex and age. Therefore, it is best to fine-tune the amount of calories appropriate to you from your weight loss and hunger levels. When losing weight, you will experience some hunger, especially before meals, but you should not be constantly hungry. If you are not losing weight and rarely hungry, then you probably need to reduce your calories, and vice versa. When weighing yourself, ideally do so upon waking, and only do it once or twice a week.

Lean Muscle to lean up

This plan has high amounts of Lean Muscle foods, such as meat, eggs, low-fat dairy, beans, protein powders and vegan alternatives. Proteins has the lowest net calories once digested and the highest satiety compared to carbs and fats, so we feel fuller on fewer calories. Protein also helps to maintain muscle as we lose weight, keeping our metabolic rate higher.

It is certainly possible to lose fat on a low-protein diet, but fat loss has consistently been shown to be more effective with a diet that contains a good amount of protein, in the range of 1.6–2.2g per kg of bodyweight per day.

Health keeps hunger at bay

The enemy of any fat-loss plan is to be constantly hungry. Therefore, the plan uses three main meals throughout the day and one snack; however, we are still limiting calories, so we need to get the biggest bang for our buck from the food that we eat. Eating meals designated as high in Health ensures that we are nutritionally fulfilled, which dampens hunger signals and keeps the body functioning optimally. Fibre, which is found in high amounts in foods such as vegetables, wholegrains and fruit, makes us feel full and isn't digested as energy, and so it is great for fat loss. Fibre is also key for gut health, which has been shown to be important in weight control. Meals high in Health also boost energy levels and metabolism, and they support our immune system, which can be challenged during fat-loss periods. We need to *prioritise* foods that are high in Health and low in calories; *moderate* the foods that are high in Health and high in calories; and *limit* foods that are low in Health and high in calories, as illustrated in the graphic overleaf.

Fluctuate your fuel

Carbs get an undeserved bad rap when it comes to losing fat, mainly as a result of misinformed social media posts and the recent prominence of keto diets. Keto diets restrict carb intake to very low levels (normally less than 50g per day) and principally work by reducing calorie intake, as carbs are our most common food group. The sustained low carb levels also stimulate 'ketosis', a process in which the body converts fat into ketones to be used for energy in the place of carbs, thereby increasing fat breakdown. Keto diets have been shown to be effective for weight loss and beneficial to the management of type-2 diabetes. However, keto diets are often unsustainable long term, as food choice, convenience and enjoyment are significantly restricted, and important nutrients, such as fibre, can become deficient. Also, if you exercise or take part in sport, your high-intensity exercise capacity will be significantly reduced.

A key principle of Colour-Fit is to vary your carb intake in line with your training/activity levels. The plan involves some tough training so we increase the amount of Fuel around the circuits and longer steady endurance training to support effective training, and overall health. Fuel intake is reduced on less active days. The point is not that carbs are bad for fat loss but that reducing them allows for increased Lean Muscle and Health foods that *are* good for fat loss, while moderating overall calorie intake. Fuel sources should be wholemeal grains, vegetables and fruit as these are better for our health than processed carbs. Vegans demonstrate that it is perfectly possible to lose weight while eating carbs: on average they eat more carbs and are slimmer than their non-vegan counterparts.

Calorie density (vertical axis)

Nutrient density (horizontal axis)

Ice cream

Low nutrients + high cals = eat infrequently

Cakes

Nut butters

Dark chocolate

Nuts

Seeds

Chocolate

Granola

Cheese

Dried fruits

Oats

High nutrients + high cals = eat moderately

Sweets

White bread

Brown bread

Red meat

Avocado

Oily fish

Fizzy drinks

Brown rice

Chickpeas

Eggs

White pasta

Tofu

White meat

White fish

Beans

High nutrients + low cals = eat frequently

Fruits

White potato

Skim milk

0% Greek yogurt

Sweet potato

Diet drinks

Low nutrients + low cals = eat moderately

Salads

Vegetables

Watch those late-night snacks

Netflix and chill in the evenings often translates to Netflix and treats instead. As we begin to wind down in the evening, we can interpret this as a sign that we are low on energy and soon unconsciously find ourselves tucking into convenient, and usually calorie-dense, snacks and treats. Time-restricted feeding (sometimes referred to as intermittent fasting) provides an additional rationale for avoiding late-night feeding. It involves limiting the time period over the course of the day when you take on calories, and has been shown to result in enhanced fat loss and metabolic health, mainly due to the reduction in calories consumed overall, but also from a small increase in fat burning due to sustained low insulin levels. Fasting (not consuming calories) for long periods is difficult, but as little as 13 hours has been shown to produce benefits for weight loss and health. This is easily achievable if you build your fasting period around sleep and either restrict eating for a period in the evening before or in the morning (for example, not eating after 7pm and resuming at 8am). Limiting food in the evening has been shown to produce slightly better fat loss than limiting it during the morning; probably due to matching our wake and sleep cycles and less optimal blood glucose control in the evening. Therefore, the eating plan places snacks during the day, leaving a good window before the morning fasted-endurance training.

Master your mind

Using smaller plates and bowls has been shown to reduce the amount of food needed to feel full, so avoid using large crockery. Also, taking your time when eating and chewing food thoroughly results in feeling full sooner, so intermittently put down your cutlery, have conversations and do not mindlessly scoff your food in front of the TV. Finally, our willpower can be flimsy when it comes to resisting food as we are hard-wired to consume calories (an evolutionary survival mechanism from when food was scarce), therefore it is better simply not to have certain foods in the house rather than try to resist them when they are in reach. Remember, though, food is a joy so the odd treat now and again is fine – I eat a little chocolate every day – and helps you to sustain good nutrition principles most of the time.

Muscle-growth Plan

Millions of us go to the gym or do push-ups and sit-ups at home with the intention of looking more muscular and athletic, and this plan will help to ensure that you are looking tip-top. For sports people, muscle growth is often important, as strength is related the muscle size and extra mass can be important in collision sports, such as American football and rugby. Women often avoid muscle-growth training for fear of looking masculine, but female hormone profiles mean that large muscle growth is rare, and therefore this programme will result in your muscles looking more toned and shapely. The plan is suitable for those who are relatively new to strength training, through to regular gym goers. An experienced strength trainer who desires large gains in muscle would need more regular, higher volume training.

Training plan: muscle growth

The aim of the training plan is to expose a wide range of muscles to strength-size training in a time-efficient manner. The plan requires the strength equipment that you would find in most gyms or well-equipped home gyms.

Feel the burn! Feel it everywhere and feel it often

Muscle growth requires regular strength-size training for a range of body parts. People often focus on the muscles they can see, such as the abs and chest, but whole-body development is needed to avoid posture problems and injury. Strength size involves using reasonably heavy weights and performing the exercises to failure level (which means you cannot do any more reps with good form). You therefore expose the muscle to the two main muscle-growth stimuli: high force and high metabolites, such as lactic acid, so you 'feel the burn'. The sets and repetitions are mainly in the strength-size range (3–6 sets of 6–10 reps) but they sometimes start in the strength-endurance range and progress to the strength-max range, for safe progression and a varied muscle stimulus (the rationale for this is explained in the training principles section on pages 203–4). We also use techniques such as reverse pyramids to increase metabolic build-up: this involves reducing the weight/resistance slightly each set but resting only a short time (20–30 seconds) before performing the next set. The minimal rest results in a build-up of metabolites which stimulate muscle growth. Sets and reps are shown as sets × reps, or a sequence of numbers that indicates the number of reps for each set (for example 8-6-6 would indicate 8 reps for the first set and 6 reps for the next 2 sets).

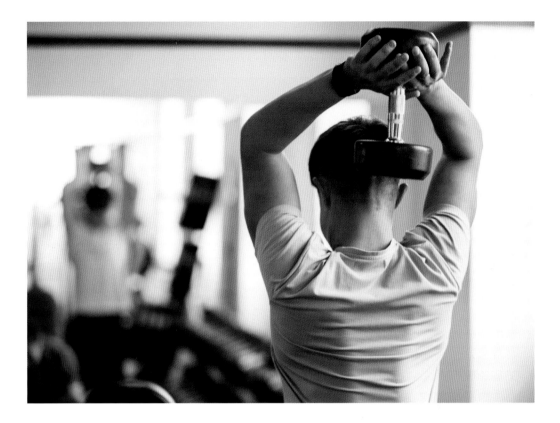

The plan involves two sessions that are ideally performed twice each per week. If you are a novice to strength training, you can still get good results from performing each session once a week, but twice is still better. To train a wide range of muscles regularly, while allowing for sufficient recovery, the plan uses a split training approach that targets different body parts on different sessions. Session 1 trains legs, shoulders and arm muscles, and Session 2 trains chest, back and core muscles.

Slick session structure

The sessions start with exercises that involve large muscle groups, to better elicit muscle growth hormones which then optimise muscle growth responses for the rest of the session. Many of the exercises in the plan are performed in pairs indicated by the same number (for example 1a and 1b). For such exercises you perform the first exercise, rest a short while (say, 1 minute), and then perform the second exercise, before returning to the first exercise. The paired exercises use different muscle groups and therefore the required rest time between the sets is reduced.

SESSION 1

LEGS, SHOULDERS AND ARMS; SIZE AND SMALL AMOUNT OF MAX STRENGTH

1a Deadlift	Coaching cues	Week	Structure
	Bend to reach the bar with arms straight, back flat, chest out. Stand pushing with the legs, then drive the hips through. Reverse the movement to return weight to floor.	1	3 × 10
		2	3 × 10
		3	3 × 8
		4	3 × 8
		5	8-8-6-6
		6	8-8-6-6

1b Shoulder press	Coaching cues	Week	Structure
	Hold bar with overhand grip and lift to shoulder height. Push weight above head until arms are fully extended, reverse the movement to return barbell to shoulders.	1	3 × 10
		2	3 × 10
		3	3 × 8
		4	3 × 8
		5	4 × 6
		6	4 × 6

2a Leg press	Coaching cues	Week	Structure
	Feet flat against the pad, push the weight up through the heels until fully extended. Pause, then reverse the movement.	1	3 × 12
		2	3 × 10
		3	3 × 10
		4	Reverse pyramid: 5 x 10
		5	Reverse pyramid: 6 x 10
		6	Reverse pyramid: 6 x 10

2b Upright row	Coaching cues	Week	Structure
	Using a overhand grip, alternately raise dumbbells to chest height, keeping weight close to your body, pushing the elbows out. As the arm returns to the start position, start to raise the weight with the other arm.	1	3 × 10
		2	3 × 10
		3	3 × 8
		4	3 × 8
		5	4 × 6
		6	4 × 6

3a Step up	Coaching cues	Week	Structure
	Barbell rested on shoulders. Place a foot on an elevated surface. Push through to stand tall, then lower to the start position.	1	2 × 12 each leg
		2	2 × 12 each leg
		3	3 × 10 each leg
		4	3 × 10 each leg
		5	3 × 8 each leg
		6	3 × 8 each leg

3b Lateral raise	Coaching cues	Week	Structure
	Stand side-on to cable and grab with far arm. Laterally raise the cable with arm remaining just slightly bent, until arm is in line with shoulder. Reverse movement to return cable to hip.	1	3 × 12 each arm
		2	3 × 12 each arm
		3	3 × 10 each arm
		4	3 × 10 each arm
		5	3 × 8 each arm
		6	3 × 8 each arm

NOTE: *Perform the same number of exercises as pairs to reduce rest (about 1 minute between each)*

SESSION 2

CHEST, BACK AND CORE; SIZE AND SMALL AMOUNT OF MAX STRENGTH

1a Decline bench	Coaching cues	Week	Structure
	Keep back flat on bench, engage core, then lower bar to chest. Press the weight up away from chest until arms are fully extended.	1	3 × 10
		2	3 × 10
		3	3 × 8
		4	3 × 8
		5	8-8-6-6
		6	8-8-6-6

1b 3-point row	Coaching cues	Week	Structure
	Back straight, engage your core, pull the weight towards your body, slightly below the shoulder. Reverse movement to return arm to full extension.	1	3 × 10 each arm
		2	3 × 10 each arm
		3	3 × 8 each arm
		4	3 × 8 each arm
		5	8-8-6-6 each arm
		6	8-8-6-6 each arm

2a DB alternate press	Coaching cues	Week	Structure
	Back flat against the bench, push one dumbbell up until the arm is straight and then lower to chest position. Repeat this action on the other arm.	1	3 × 10 each arm
		2	3 × 10 each arm
		3	3 × 8 each arm
		4	3 × 8 each arm
		5	10-8-6-6 each arm
		6	10-8-6-6 each arm

2b Hanging row	Coaching cues	Week	Structure
	Lie below the bar and grab the bar using an overhand grip. Keeping the body straight, pull yourself up to the bar until your chest touches, then reverse the movement until the arms are straight.	1	3 × TF
		2	3 × TF
		3	3 × TF
		4	3 × TF
		5	3 × TF
		6	3 × TF

3a Dips	Coaching cues	Week	Structure
	From arms fully locked out, bend your arms to lower your body until upper arms are parallel with the ground. Reverse the motion by straightening the arms.	1	3 × TF
		2	3 × TF
		3	3 × TF
		4	3 × TF with 10kg
		5	3 × TF with 10kg
		6	3 × TF with 10kg

3b Core circuit: rollout, deadbug, side bridge dips	Week	Structure
	1	3 × 10 of each
	2	3 × 10 of each
	3	3 × 10 of each
	4	3 × 12 of each
	5	3 × 12 of each
	6	3 × 12 of each

Roll out and back   Drop opposite arm and leg   Drop and return hip

NOTE: *Perform the same number of exercises as pairs to reduce rest (about 1 minute between each)*

TF = to fatigue

Meal plan: muscle growth

	Monday	Tuesday	Wednesday
	Training Muscle growth session 1 Training load Moderate Rationale High calories, Lean Muscle and Fuel; a focus around training	Training Rest day Training load n/a Rationale Neutral calories through less snacking; high in Lean Muscle and Health	Training Muscle growth session 2 Training load Moderate Rationale High calories, Lean Muscle and Fuel; a focus around training
Breakfast	Smoked Salmon and Guacamole Toast (page 44)	Avocado Baked Eggs (page 47	Carrot Cake Overnight Oats (page 36)
Morning snack	Almond and Berry Balls (page 163)	No snack	Ham-wrapped asparagus
Lunch	Tuna salad sandwich (see Wrap and Sandwich builder page 82)	Pea, Watercress and Carrot Salad (page 143)	Sushi Rolls (page 155)
Afternoon snack	Protein Frappuccino (page 187)	Nuts, seeds and Greek yogurt	Post-Workout Peanut Butter Blast (page 184)
Dinner	Doner Kebab and Roasted Vegetables (pages 126 and 149)	Almond-Breaded Chicken Strips, Salt and Pepper Sweet Potato Chips and Balsamic Kale (pages 72, 146 and 144)	Salmon, Tomato and Asparagus Bake (page 98)
Evening snack	Overnight oats and protein-powder porridge (see Overnight Oats Meal Builder page 56)	No snack	Crackers and cottage cheese

The key nutrition principle of the muscle-growth plan is that it has a high proportion of Lean Muscle and Performance Fuel meals. It also contains a relatively high number of calories as a result of regular snacks and the inclusion of more calorie-dense foods in meals. You'll find some guiding principles at the end of the plan on page 242.

Thursday	Friday	Saturday	Sunday
Training Rest day Training load n/a Rationale Neutral calories through less snacking; high in Lean Muscle and Health	Training Muscle growth session 1 Training load Moderate Rationale High calories, Lean Muscle and Fuel; focus around training	Training Rest day Training load n/a Rationale Neutral calories through less snacking; high in Lean Muscle and Health	Training Muscle growth session 2 Training load Moderate Rationale High in calories, Lean Muscle and Fuel; focus around training
Breakfast Baustis (page 53)	Sweet Potato Hash (page 54)	Mocha Parfait (page 30)	Healthy English Breakfast (page 51)
No snack	Almond Cobbler (page 157)	No snack	Smoked salmon and antipasti
Beef-Stuffed Peppers (page 120)	Peanut Butter and Banana Wrap (page 77)	Huevos Rancheros (page 88)	Grilled Halloumi Wrap (page 79)
Mocha Parfait (page 30)	Whey protein shake (see Smoothie Builder, page 192)	Peanut butter and celery	Beef jerky
Steak, baked new potatoes and asparagus	Power Paella (page 103)	Chinese Beef Noodles (page 123)	Healthy Chicken Pie, Cajun Street Rice and steamed veg (pages 115 and 140)
No snack	Lean Crêpe (page 41)	No snack	Rice pudding pot

Some guiding principles

Consume those calories

We are best able to gain muscle when we consume a positive calorie balance over a sustained period, which is why this meal plan has three meals a day plus three snacks on training days and one or two snacks on non-training days. A calorie surplus of about 10 per cent is thought to be optimal so that we have extra energy to generate new muscular tissue while not having an excess that would be converted to fat. Novice trainers can actually gain muscle on a negative calorie balance, but muscle growth is always more optimal with a positive calorie balance. On days where there is no strength training, calories are reduced so as not to promote fat gain, and the Health element increased because of its importance to overall well-being.

Lean Muscle = lean muscle

The meal plan consistently contains meals high in Lean Muscle. Proteins are the building blocks of muscle. Muscle growth is optimised by providing protein feeds of roughly 20–40g every 3–4 hours during the day, but as long as you are having 1.6–2g per kg of your bodyweight over the day, muscle growth will be well supported. Do not fear if you are vegan, you can easily attain sufficient protein for optimum muscle growth by consuming a range of beans, pulses, wholegrains, soya products such as tofu, tempeh and dairy substitutes, and mycoprotein or meat substitutes.

Bedtime snacks in the plan have a greater proportion of casein protein (often found in dairy products), which is a slow-release protein that will drip-feed muscles during the night, leading to less muscle loss during this fasting period. The use of protein supplements, particularly those that are high in the amino acid leucine, such as whey, are advised for strength training, as they are rapidly absorbed into the muscular tissue, and leucine has a stronger muscle-building effect than other amino acids. Many vegan protein powders also exist that are well absorbed and have a good leucine content.

'Fuel' muscle growth

Fuel consumption is important around training to supply the high-intensity energy required for strength training and to stimulate muscle-growth hormones, such as insulin. Regular fuel consumption also ensures that we are consuming sufficient calories. The uptake of carbs in the muscle also draws in water (3g of water for every 1g of carbs), which increases muscle size.

Running Plan, Middle Distance

(10km to half marathon)

Running is the most popular form of keeping fit, and millions of us compete in races, from park run 5km, right up to marathons and ultrarunning. If you would like to perform well in a middle-distance event, such as 10km up to a half marathon, this plan will boost your performance to new heights. The plan will help you perform to your best, rather than just complete the distance, so you'll need to be reasonably fit and committed to training. If you do not have the time or fitness levels to complete all the training, completing the Tuesday, Friday and Sunday sessions will still get you in great shape to perform well for the big race.

Training Plan: running plan, middle distance

Go far and fast

Middle distances are aptly described as in the 'middle' of the intensity spectrum. They are quite long but short enough so that good runners can push the pace to around anaerobic threshold throughout (see explanation on page 197). Therefore, this programme mainly consists of aerobic training with a good proportion involving threshold endurance running. It includes regular higher intensity methods, such as max aerobic, as they are so effective at improving performance. The training plan is for about three months and progressively increases the overall training load and the amount of higher intensity running. Where a range is given, gradually increase your training duration through the weeks as you feel fitter.

The longer you train, the longer you taper

This training plan is slightly longer than most in the book. The longer the training period and the longer the event distance, the longer the taper period needs to be due to the greater stresses the body goes through. Therefore, the plan has two weeks of reduced training load for the final phase, with the inclusion of lower volume, higher intensity training so that fitness stays high. Some low-intensity training is also used to keep the legs ticking over, but with a low overall load. Training intensity is indicated by the colours explained in the key at the bottom of the plan overleaf.

RUNNING SCHEDULE, MIDDLE DISTANCE

Phase	Monday	Tuesday	Wednesday
Weeks 1–3: prepare	Steady ~30–35 minutes	Threshold – 3 × ~8–10 minutes	Rest day
Training Load Gauge			
Weeks 4–6: build	Steady ~40–60 minutes	Threshold 2 × ~15 minutes	Rest day
Training Load Gauge			
Weeks 7–9: specific	Steady ~20 minutes Max intervals @ ~95% 10 × 30 seconds, 1½ minutes rest	Threshold ~30 minutes	Rest day
Training Load Gauge			
Weeks 10–11: taper/race	Threshold ~2 × 8 minutes Max intervals 95% 5 × 30 seconds, 1 minute rest	Rest day	Max aerobic 3 × 3 minutes, 1½ minutes rest
Training Load Gauge			

Thursday	Friday	Saturday	Sunday
Steady ~30–35 minutes	Max aerobic 5 × 3 minutes, 1½ minutes rest	Rest day	Steady ~20 minutes Max intervals @ ~90% 6 × 1 minute, 2 minutes easy
Steady ~40–60 minutes	Max aerobic 4 × 4 minutes, 2 minutes rest	Rest day	Threshold 2 × 12 minutes Max intervals @ ~95% 8 × 30 seconds, 1½ minutes rest
Steady ~40–60 minutes	Max Aaerobic 5 × 3½> minutes, 2 minutes rest	Rest day	~¾ to full race distance
Rest day	Steady ~20–40 minutes	Rest day	Week 10: ~ ½ to ¾ race distance Week 11: race

Training bar key: ● steady ○ threshold ◐ max aerobic ● max intervals ◉ mixed training

Abbreviations: ~ approximately

Meal plan: running plan, middle distance

Fuel the performance fire

The plan involves regular training, with the aim of pushing yourself in order to improve fitness. Performance Fuel and sufficient calories are therefore key components of the meal plan,

	Monday	Tuesday	Wednesday
	Training Morning, extensive Training load Moderate Rationale Fuel emphasised prior to the run, balanced after	Training Afternoon, threshold Training load Moderate to hard Rationale Fuel bias for most of the day for intense training	Training Rest Training load n/a Rationale Focus on Health and Lean Muscle, but some Fuel for Thursday's run
Breakfast	Apple and Date Bircher (page 31)	Almond and Banana Pancakes (page 39)	Breakfast Burrito (page 39)
Morning snack	Walnut Chocolate Truffles (page 168)	No snack	No snack
Lunch	Peanut Butter and Banana Wrap (page 77)	Tabbouleh (page 138)	Chilli con Carne (page 119)
Afternoon snack	No snack	Mango and Orange Smoothie (page 190)	Joint Jellies (page 160)
Dinner	Healthy Chicken Pie and Roasted Veg (pages 115 and 149)	Beef Stroganoff (page 121)	Autumn Chicken and Veggie Bake (page 109)
Evening snack	No snack	Greek yogurt sprinkled with cocoa	No snack

with three main meals and between one and three snacks per day. On rest days, Performance Fuel and overall calories are reduced, but still play an important role, to optimise your fuel stores for the next day's training. Health is also a key consideration and there is a Health component, such as fruit and vegetables, in many of the meals. Lean Muscle is also an important component and is emphasised following training, to aid recovery.

Thursday	Friday	Saturday	Sunday
Training Morning, extensive Training load Moderate Rationale Fuel prioritised for upcoming race	Training Afternoon, max aerobic Training load Hard Rationale Fuel bias in afternoon; Lean Muscle post run	Training Rest Training load n/a Rationale Balanced to promote Health and Lean Muscle, but some Fuel for Sunday run	Training Morning, race practice Training load Hard Rationale Fuel for run; then Fuel and Lean Muscle post run
Mango and Banana Parfait (page 30)	Huevos Rancheros (page 88)	Healthy English Breakfast (page 51)	Vanilla and Blueberry Overnight Oats (page 38)
No snack	No snack	No snack	Banana Bread (page 175)
Lemon Pasta with Courgette and Tomato (page 85)	Mango and Pineapple Salad (page 65)	Easy Tuna Salad (page 68)	Tuna salad wholemeal sub (see Wrap and Sandwich Builder page 82) and milk
Beetroot and Mixed Berry Smoothie (page 185)	Blueberry and Banana Oat Muffins (page 176)	Avocado Brownies (page 171)	Joint Panna Cotta (page 177)
Power Paella (page 103)	Vegan Sausages and Salt and Pepper Sweet Potato Chips (pages 96 and 146)	Moussaka (page 128)	Turkey Bolognese (page 114)
No snack	Porridge	Toast	No snack

Sprint Triathlon Plan

Sometimes we can get stuck in a rut with training and it becomes a bit stale. I found that an awesome way to spice things up is to train for a triathlon. I'm sure many of you, like me, will initially find the prospect of a triathlon a bit daunting but a great way to start is with a sprint triathlon, where you typically swim 750m, bike 20km and run 5km. The different fitness disciplines (cycling, swimming and running) provided new challenges, and the 'off-load' nature of cycling and swimming helped my ageing joints. In the end I was hooked and with the help of this plan I'm sure you will love it too.

This plan is designed for anyone with reasonable fitness levels who wants to perform well. Even this shortest form of triathlon is pretty tough and it requires regular training, with some double sessions so that you get used to the transition demands of triathlon.

Training plan: sprint triathlon

My friend Rob Harvey helped me design the triathlon plan. He has trained Olympic, world and Commonwealth triathlon champions, such as the Brownlee brothers and Non Stanford, and is an even bigger hero for overcoming a rare form of cancer. The principal aim of the training is to perform all the triathlon disciplines at least once per week, using mainly moderate- to higher-intensity endurance methods. The plan lasts two months and requires access to a bike and a pool or open water. If you are limited for time, perform the sessions on a Tuesday, Thursday and Sunday. Maximal aerobic and maximal interval training should be preceded by a short warm-up.

Push and progress

Sprint triathlons are short enough to push yourself throughout. Therefore, training involves the range of endurance methods but mainly threshold training. To establish a good fitness base, and to progress safely, the plan uses extensive steady training more towards the start of the programme. Maximal aerobic training is used intermittently throughout, as it is a powerful performance stimulus for endurance events. The swimming section is relatively short, so we use some maximal intervals in the pool. Overall training load is progressed through the programme, except for the final week when there is a reduction in overall training load so that you are super-fit and fresh for the big day.

Train transitions

Triathlons require sequential performance of the swim, bike and run components. It can feel a bit weird quickly switching from one form of exercise to another, and critical minutes can be lost putting on the different footwear and apparel, if you are not well practised. Therefore, the programme on the following pages contains some sessions where you perform two different disciplines. In the penultimate phase of the programme it's recommended that you try to recreate the demands of the race, if possible.

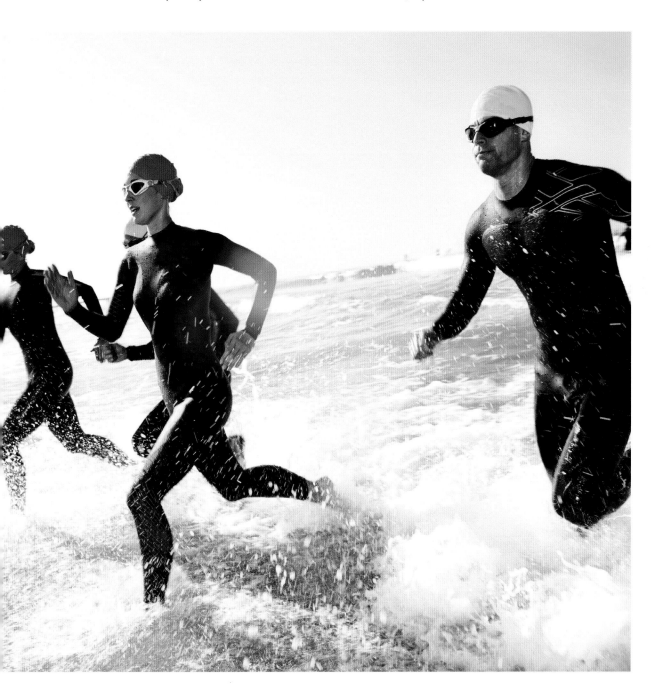

SPRINT TRIATHLON SCHEDULE

Phase	Monday	Tuesday	Wednesday
Weeks 1–2: prepare	Rest day	**Swim** Steady ~10 minutes Threshold ~3 × 5 minutes, 1 minute rest	**Bike** Threshold ~2 × 15 minutes, 2 minutes slow recovery
Training Load Gauges			
Weeks 3–4: build	Rest day	**Swim** Steady ~10 minutes Threshold ~3 × 6 minutes, 1 minute rest	**Bike** Threshold/hilly route ~45 minutes
Training Load Gauges			
Weeks 5–7: specific	Rest day	**Swim** Threshold ~4 × 5 minutes, 1 minute rest **Run** Max aerobic ~4 × 4 minutes, 2 minutes rest	**Bike** Threshold/hilly route ~45 minutes
Training Load Gauges			
Week 8: taper/race	Rest day	**Swim** Threshold ~3 × 5 minutes, 1 minute rest	**Bike** Threshold ~20–30 minutes
Training Load Gauges			

Thursday	Friday	Saturday	Sunday
Run Max aerobic ~5 × 2 minutes, 1 minute rest	Rest day	**Bike** Steady ~ 60 minutes	**Swim** Steady ~10 minutes, max interval 15 × ~25m, 45 seconds rest
			Run Threshold ~2 × 10 minutes, 2 minutes slow rest
Run Steady ~10 minutes Max aerobic ~4 × 3 minutes, 90 seconds rest	Rest day	**Run** Threshold ~3 × 10 minutes, 1 minute slow recovery	**Swim** Max interval 20 × ~25 minutes, 30 seconds rest
			Bike Steady ~60–80 minutes
Run Max interval ~10 × 20 seconds @ 90%, 40 seconds rest	Rest day	**Bike** Threshold ~ 20 minutes	**Practice race** Perform specific discipline of the race and sequence together if possible to practise transitions
		Swim Threshold ~2 x 10 minutes, 1 minute rest	
Run Max aerobic ~2 × 4 minutes, 2 minutes rest	Rest day	**Bike** Steady ~ 20 minutes	Race day

Training bar key: ● steady ● threshold ● max aerobic ● max intervals ● mixed training

Abbreviations: ~ approximately

Meal plan: sprint triathlon

The meal plan below is for one week. All the weeks of the programme, except the final week, follow a similar training structure so the plan provides a suitable meal structure for the vast majority of the programme. (Some guiding principles, and advice for the final week, can be found on page 254.)

	Monday	Tuesday	Wednesday
	Training Rest day Training load n/a Rationale Health and Lean Muscle is the focus for most meals	Training Morning swim Training load Moderate Rationale Slight emphasis on Fuel for moderate training load	Training Afternoon bike Training load Moderate Rationale Slight emphasis on Fuel for moderate training load
Breakfast	Green Shakshuka (page 55)	Chocolate Orange Pancakes (page 42)	Breakfast Burrito (page 39)
Morning snack	No snack	Pear or apple	No snack
Lunch	Mediterranean Wrap (page 76)	Loaded But Light Potato Skins (page 141)	Spanish Tomato Salad (page 69)
Afternoon snack	Apple or pear	No snack	Antipasti
Dinner	Thai Fishcakes and Roasted Vegetables (pages 106 and 149)	Beef Stroganoff (page 121)	Fish Pie (page 104)
Evening snack	No snack	Mocha Parfait (page 30)	Lean Crêpe (page 41)

Thursday	Friday	Saturday	Sunday
Training Afternoon run **Training load** Hard **Rationale** Fuel bias; Lean Muscle at night to aid recovery	**Training** Rest day **Training load** n/a **Rationale** Health and Lean Muscle focus in morning but Fuel included later for hard training tomorrow	**Training** Morning run **Training load** Moderate **Rationale** Fuel around morning for harder training	**Training** Morning swim/bike **Training load** Hard **Rationale** Fuel around morning for harder training
Kiwi and Banana Parfait (page 33)	Healthy Mexican Eggs (page 48)	Vanilla and Blueberry Overnight Oats (page 38)	Apple and Date Bircher (page 31)
No snack	No snack	Banana	Apricot and Dark Chocolate Fuel Bars (page 166)
Ham, Egg and Avocado Wrap (page 77)	Easy Tuna Salad (page 68)	Grilled Halloumi Wrap (page 79)	Chilli con Carne (page 119)
Trail mix and Greek yogurt	Edamame Summer Rolls (page 158)	Lean Strawberry Smoothie (page 188)	Joint Panna Cotta (page 177)
Lamb Kefta, Salt and Pepper Sweet Potato Chips (pages 125 and 146) and peas	Autumn Chicken and Veggie Bake (page 109)	Aubergine and Lentil Bake (page 87)	Rapid Chicken Sunday Dinner (page 166)
Hot milk and biscuits	No snack	Greek yogurt and blueberries	No snack

Some guiding principles

Lots of training = lots of fuelling and recovery

The training plan requires some regular tough training, with some double sessions, so the meal plan typically has three main meals and two snacks per day to support calories needs. The plan has a relatively high proportion of Performance Fuel meals and increases fuel intake around tougher training to maximise performance. On rest days, fuel is reduced, as physical demands are lower, and to promote Health and Lean Muscle foods which will support the immune system and help you to stay lean.

Lean Muscle is emphasised in addition to fuel post-training to restore carb stores and hasten muscle recovery. The macro guide on page 212 provides some further guidance as to the amount of carbs, protein and fat we should be aiming to consume based on our training and goals.

Top-up during your taper week

As with most sport performance programmes, the final week(s) involves a taper period, where overall training is reduced so you are as fresh as possible for the big day. Although training is reduced, Fuel should remain a consistent feature with relatively balanced meals throughout the week. Around 1–2 days before the event (longer for harder events) you should increase the proportion of Fuel to maximise fuel stores and performance potential. On the day of the event, you want to be fuelled but feel light and have an empty stomach to avoid gastric problems. Therefore, some foods we would not normally encourage are acceptable, such as white versions of breads and pasta, and sugary confectionery and beverages, as they are high-carb, light and digested quickly. Avoid fatty foods as they slow digestion. Have your final meal around 3 hours before the event when possible and consume only light snacks and drinks close to the event.

Cycle 100 Plan

I absolutely love mountain-biking around the beautiful Peak District, but the lure of Lycra to a middle-aged man is irresistible, so I've found myself road biking more and more. Cycling is a great form of exercise that is easy on the joints, gets us outside and is a gloriously green form of transportation. London 100 is one of the most popular races in the world and, as you can guess, involves cycling 100 miles as fast as possible. No easy task! This plan would also be suitable for any cycle enduro event.

To design the plan, I enlisted the help of one my best pals, Ben Leach, who is one of the UK's premier physical trainers and rides for Team Onyx. This plan will help you to compete at your best in just 12 weeks. It requires a reasonable level of cycling fitness, but by no means elite, and a good commitment to training. If you are limited for training time, performing the training on Tuesday, Thursday and Sunday will still get you good results. Unsurprisingly, the plan requires access to a bike and relevant equipment. Access to a stationary Wattbike or similar is handy for the interval training but not essential. The strength training requires access to equipment found in most gyms.

Training plan: cycle 100, endurance

One hundred miles is a long way! A competent rider would require about 6 hours if riding in a group, or 7 hours if riding on their own (riding in a group gives improved aerodynamics). Such extensive exercise durations dictate that the plan focuses on extensive steady training, especially on weekends when people tend to have more time. Initially, we use moderately long, steady sessions on both weekend days, but as the plan progresses we concentrate on single, longer efforts to prepare for race conditions. Threshold and max aerobic training also feature regularly and are progressed throughout the plan, as they are proficient in eliciting aerobic adaptations that supply energy for sustained periods.

Push the pace

Cycle races are seldom done at the same pace throughout. Cyclists frequently have phasic bursts where they push hard to break away from, or catch, a group, or for a sprint finish. Similarly, race routes are rarely flat and frequently feature many hills and even mountains. Therefore, we need to train to push ourselves hard for different periods of the race, so the plan uses max intervals training after developing a solid aerobic base, and it has a focus on power endurance towards the latter part of the programme. Both the max aerobic and max interval sessions should be preceded by a steady 5-minute warm-up.

Cycle geeks!

Many cyclists obsess over data and power output, which can be accurately measured using modern bike equipment and apps. Gauging real-time power output enables an accurate assessment of training intensity based on performance tests, the most common in cycling being functional threshold power (FTP). FTP is very similar to the threshold test of average power over 20 minutes but with a 5 per cent reduction. If you are accustomed to using FTP, the approximate ranges for the other types of training are shown in the table below.

Training method	% FTP
Steady	70–90%
Threshold	95–105%
Max aerobic	110–120%
Max intervals	
~90%	~140–155%
~95%	~160–170%

All the gear ...

Many a time I've been slogging away and a cyclist has cruised past me barely pedalling! The mantra 'aero is everything' is a commonplace in cycling. A good bike, helmet and clips, and proper fitting garments, can greatly enhance your aerodynamics and speed. A lower aero position (bent forward at the hips so your head is lower) is often desirable for good aerodynamics, and we provide a simple yoga programme to help you achieve this and reduce the stress on your back and neck muscles by improving your hip and upper-back mobility.

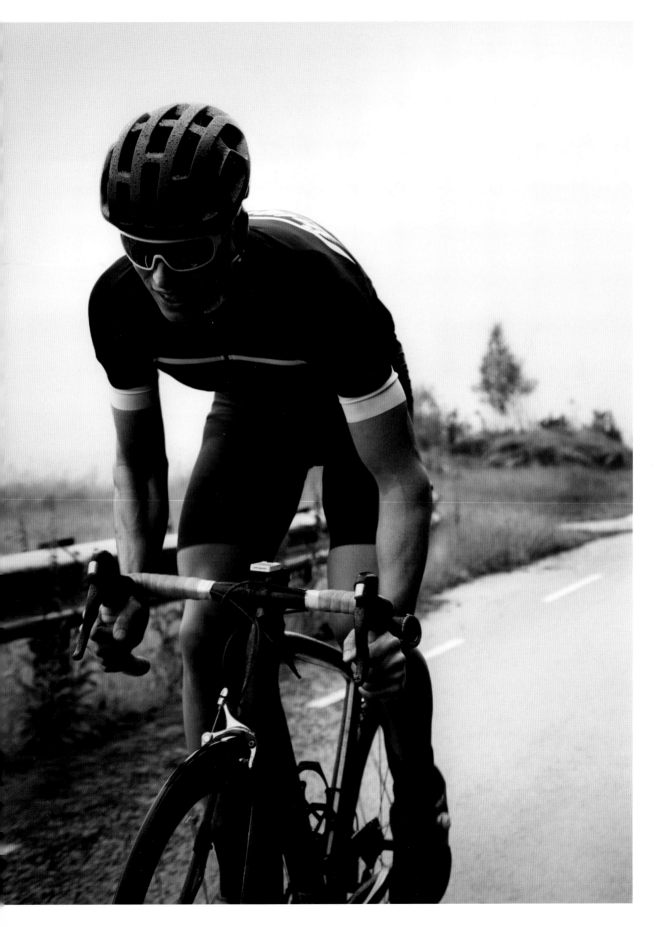

CYCLE 100 SCHEDULE

Phase	Monday	Tuesday	Wednesday
Weeks 1–2: base endurance		Threshold ~30 minutes	Strength and yoga session
Training Load Gauges	Rest day		
Weeks 3–4: build endurance		Threshold ~40 minutes	Strength and yoga session
Training Load Gauges	Rest day		
Weeks 5–6: efficiency		Threshold ~50 minutes	Strength and yoga session
Training Load Gauges	Rest day		
Weeks 7–8: max aerobic		Max intervals @ ~90% max 20 × 30 seconds, 60 seconds steady in between	Strength and yoga session
Training Load Gauges	Rest day		
Week 9–10: power endurance		Max intervals @ ~95% max 30 × 15 seconds, 45 seconds steady in between	Strength and yoga session
Training Load Gauges	Rest day		
Week 11: maintain		Max intervals @ ~90% max 30 × 30 seconds, 30 seconds steady in between	Strength and yoga session
Training Load Gauges	Rest day		
Week 12: taper		Threshold ~30 minutes	Yoga session
Training Load Gauges	Rest day		

Training bar key: ● steady ● threshold max aerobic ● max intervals mixed training

Abbreviations: ~ approximately

Thursday	Friday	Saturday	Sunday
Max aerobic 5 × 3 minutes, 2 minutes steady in between	Rest day	Steady ~1 hour	Steady ~1½ hours
Max aerobic 4 × 4 minutes, 2 minutes steady in between	Rest day	Steady ~1 hour	Steady ~2 hours
Max aerobic Pyramid 4/3/2/1/2/3/4 minutes, with equal steady rest in between	Rest day	Steady ~1 hour	Steady ~2½ hours
Max aerobic pyramid 4/3/2/1/2/3/4 minutes, with equal steady rest in between	Rest day	Threshold ~45 minutes	Steady ~3½ hours
Max intervals @ ~90% max 16 × 60 seconds, 60 seconds steady in between	Rest day	Threshold ~45 minutes	Steady ~5–6 hours
Max aerobic 4 × 4 minutes, 2 minutes steady in between	Rest day	Threshold ~1 hour	Steady ~2 hours
Max aerobic 3 × 3 minutes, 2 minutes steady in between	Rest day	Race	Rest/Party

Strength Training

Cycling is basically a repeated leg-pushing event, so improving our leg strength can significantly improve our cycling ability. Core strength is also important to resist rotational forces, generate power when standing and to cope with the postural strains of cycling. As this is a long event, improving economy is key. This is best achieved using strength-max training as it maximally increases strength without putting on much muscle mass, so each pedal becomes easier. Some initial strength-size training is used to lay the foundations to optimally increase strength. The volume of strength training is reduced in weeks 9–11 because of a steep increase in volume from the cycling training. There is no strength training in the final week to optimise freshness for the big day. Strength-endurance training is not considered important, because the normal cycling training will induce similar adaptations.

Yoga plan

This simple yoga programme can be done before or after the strength training and whenever desired, as it has a minimal training load. Perform the exercises in sequence, holding for 20–30 seconds and repeat 1–4 times.

Upward dog	Downward dog	Warrior one
Inhale as you straighten your arms and extend your spine. Exhale attempting to keep your hips on the floor and extending the strech further.	Inhale as you lift your hips. Exhale and try to achieve a straight line through your legs and trunk/arms. Bend at knee slightly if struggling to keep back staight.	In a lunge position, aim to have the back foot flat and leg straight. Inhale and reach up, lifting the shoulder blades and arching the back. Exhale and try to stretch the hips and back/arms further.

SESSION 1

LEGS AND CORE

Alternate the same-numbered exercise. Rest 90 seconds per exercise

* see page 234 for explanation of sequence of numbers used for reps

1a Back squat	Coaching cues	Week	Structure
	Stand with the bar on your upper back. Keeping heels down, back straight and knees aligned, squat down, moving the hips back as if sitting. Aim for thighs to be parallel to ground and return to the start position.	1–2	3 × 8
		3–5	4 × 6
		6–8	6-5-4-4*
		9–11	6-4

1b Kneeling woodchop	Coaching cues	Week	Structure
	Ideally use a cable, but any weight can work. Kneel in lunge with leg nearest to cable on the floor. Move the weight diagonally up across the body and return. Keep back upright and aim to rotate with upper back so that lower back is stable.	1–2	3 × 10
		3–5	3 × 10
		6–8	3 × 8
		9–11	8-7-6*

2a Step-up	Coaching cues	Week	Structure
	Barbell resting on shoulders, or hold dumbbells, place a foot on an elevated surface so that the thigh is almost parallel to the ground. Place your weight on elevated foot and push through to stand tall, then lower to the start position. 3 minutes rest per set.	1–2	3 × 8
		3–5	3 × 6
		6–8	6-5-4-4*
		9–11	2 × 5

2b Core circuit: perform core exercises back to back. 3 sets (alternating sets with step-up)

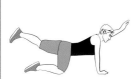

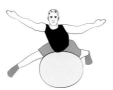

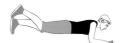

4-point extension

Straighten and elongate opposite arm and leg, and hold 4 × 5 seconds

Back extension

Bend at hips over a raised surface and return to straight position rotating arms out

10–12 reps

plank with leg raise

In a plank, raise 1 leg and hold for 2 seconds. Alternate legs 8–10 reps each side

Meal plan: cycle 100

The meal plan features one week of meals that are suitable for the training plan. The key principles are to supply fuel to support training while promoting fat as an energy source when appropriate, and to promote being lean and healthy. You'll find some guiding principles following the plan on page 264.

	Monday	Tuesday	Wednesday
	Training Rest Training load n/a Rationale Emphasis on Lean Muscle and Health, with reduced meal frequency	Training Afternoon, max intervals Training load Hard Rationale Balanced as training load is moderate	Training Afternoon, strength Training load Moderate Rationale Lean Muscle and Health take priority
Breakfast	Avocado Baked Eggs (page 47)	Chocolate Orange Pancakes (page 42)	Breakfast Baustis (page 53)
Morning snack	No snack	No snack	No snack
Lunch	Asian-Style Super-Salad (page 64)	Wraps (see Wrap and Sandwich Meal Builder, page 82)	Prawn and Asparagus Stir-Fry (page 71)
Afternoon snack	Joint Jellies (page 160)	Trail mix	Beef jerky
Dinner	Healthy Chicken Pie (page 115), new potatoes and asparagus	Turkey Burger in a bun, Salt and Pepper Sweet Potato Wedges (pages 118 and 146) and peas	Fish Pie (page 104)
Evening snack	No snack	Healthy Eton Mess (page 178)	Whey protein shake with milk (see Smoothie Builder, page 192)

Thursday	Friday	Saturday	Sunday
Training Afternoon, max aerobic Training load Hard Rationale Balanced but increased Fuel around training	Training Rest Training load n/a Rationale Health and Lean Muscle are promoted but some Fuel included	Training Morning, steady Training load Moderate to light Rationale Low morning Fuel to promote fat adaptation; balanced thereafter	Training Morning, steady Training load Very hard Rationale Fuel needed prior and during ride; Fuel and Lean Muscle post ride
Porridge with fruit	Healthy Mexican Eggs (page 48)	Poached eggs, smoked salmon and spinach	Carrot Cake Overnight Oats (page 36)
No snack	No snack	Banana and Date Flapjacks (page 172)	Mango and Coconut Balls (page 165)
Light But Loaded Potato Skins (page 141)	Tuscan Bean Soup (page 62)	Ham, Egg and Avocado Wrap (page 77)	Spicy Prawns with Quinoa (page 97)
Apple	Antipasti	No snack	Almond Cobbler (page 157)
Roasted Vegetable Lasagne (page 92)	Basil Pesto Gnocchi (page 151)	Almond-Breaded Chicken Strips and Cajun Street Rice (pages 71 and 140)	Rapid Chicken Sunday Dinner (page 116)
Lean Crêpe (page 41)	No snack	Toast (see Toast Toppers Meal Builder, page 58)	No snack

Some guiding principles

Fuel and fat

One hundred miles requires lots of training and therefore the plan frequently features meals and snacks that emphasise Performance Fuel and higher calorie loads. It includes several meals and snacks per day; however, when performing such long-duration events, it is advantageous to maximise energy from fat because we have potentially far greater reserves of energy from fat, and it spares our precious carb reserves that allow us to go faster. Therefore, some of the steady sessions that have a moderate training load do not have a high Fuel component before training as this will make us more proficient at using fat for energy. Promoting fat utilisation will also help us to stay lean. Meals and snacks around high-intensity and harder training-load sessions always have a higher Performance Fuel element to maximise performance and training adaptations.

The road to recovery, and the power:weight ratio

Lean Muscle meals and snacks feature strongly after hard training and strength training to facilitate recovery and muscle development, while Health-biased meals come more to the fore on rest days to help us stay lean and healthy. Being lean is considered extremely important in cycling, especially for longer distance events. We need to transport our bodyweight on a bike, so reducing weight, ideally through body fat, increases our power:weight ratio, making us quicker and more efficient.

Super-supplements

Up until now, I have avoided mentioning supplements, as I believe in a food-first approach; however, when it comes to performing your best in long-distance cycling events, supplements can definitely help. Carb drinks simultaneously boost hydration and fuel and so are great, but you will be limited as to how much you can carry. Drinks that are about 6–10% carbs with a glucose/maltodextrin and fructose combination are optimal. Gels are also great as they are lightweight and contain 20–40g of rapidly digested carbs. When pushing hard in a race over 2 hours, consuming about 60–90g of carbs per hour is optimal through a mix of drinks, gels and snacks. However, this requires practise and you should always rehearse your supplement strategy several times before a race, so you know it works for you and your guts become accustomed to it. Taking on this amount of carbs without practising, will definitely result in some unwanted toilet breaks!

Skill-Based Endurance Sport Plan

(football, rugby, hockey, basketball, and so on)

If you are one of the millions of us that partake in skill-based endurance sports such as football, rugby, hockey, tennis, basketball and Aussie rules, this could be the plan to take your game to the next level. To help design the plans I enlisted Jon Williams, who has been the Welsh and Lion's Rugby nutritionist for nearly 20 years. Combine that with my 20-plus years working in pro football, and you're in good hands. The plan covers the pre-season period, which is considered the key time for physical development. Therefore, it is physically demanding and suitable for keen amateurs right through to professionals. If you play more for fun or are a beginner, then training on Tuesdays and Thurdays, in addition to playing your matches at the weekend, would be more than sufficient.

Training: skill-based endurance sport

The training plan is for six weeks, which is a typical length for pre-season preparations. Skill-based endurance sports require a range of fitness qualities, therefore the programme includes both endurance and strength training.

Endurance training

The principal aim of the endurance training is to work on a range of fitness qualities progressively, while building up match fitness and simultaneously improving skills and tactics. Sounds easy!

Jack of all fitness trades

Field sports involve a range of different exercise intensities, from walking right through to maximum sprinting and rapid change of direction. Competition is prolonged and has intermittent periods of high intensity, which are key to performance so optimal training needs to utilise a range of different endurance-training methods. The plan starts with predominantly lower intensity methods and gradually increases the use of higher intensity methods. Some high intensity methods are used early on, but the proportion of their use increases as we progress. Overall training load also increases through the weeks until the final week, when it is reduced so that you start the competition season as fresh and as fit as possible. Practice competitions are commonplace in the pre-season period and they are placed on most Saturdays in the plan. It is wise to progress gradually during the duration of these practice competitions up to full competition, as they normally pose the biggest injury risk.

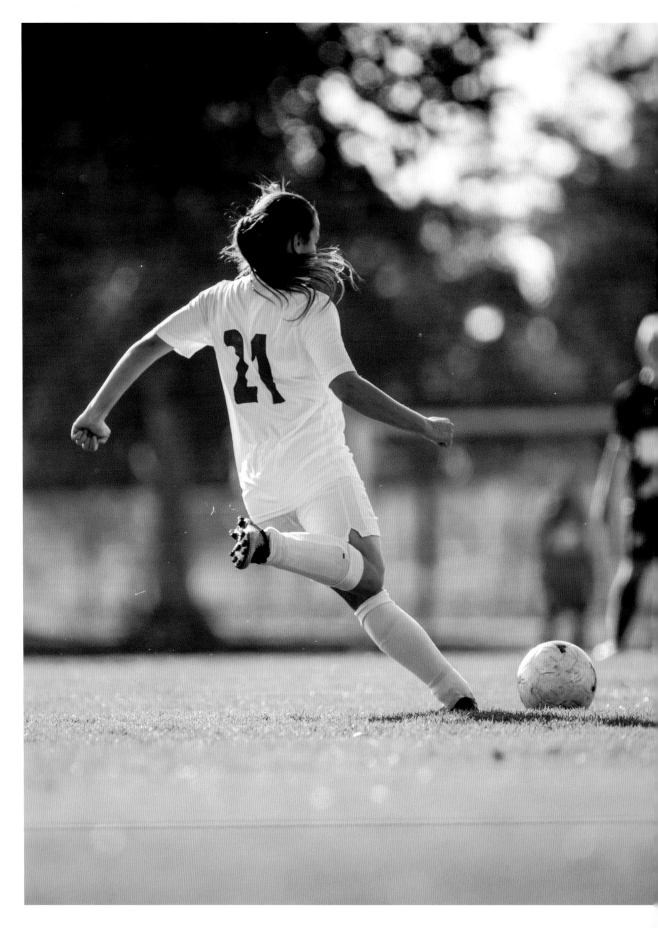

Stamina, skills and specificity in one hit

As 'skill based' infers, performance in these sports is not determined solely by fitness but also by an athlete's skill level. For this reason, skill-based sport training often uses drills that simultaneously develop skill and fitness by mimicking the demands of competition, but typically with altered team sizes and/or rules. My PhD was based on deciphering which training drills are suitable for improving different endurance training methods; the general finding being that intensity increases as the number of players in a team reduces, due to a more continual involvement in play. Furthermore, movement in skill-based sports tends to be multi-directional, with lots of non-linear movements and frequent accelerating, decelerating and turning. This means it's important for fitness drills to involve non-linear, mixed-pace running that mimics the demands of the sport. The table below shows different skill-based drills and running-based drills that can be used to train the different endurance methods, with a QR code that links to a huge range of sample training drills.

Endurance type	Skill-based drills	Running-based drills	Example drills
Steady	9–11 a side	Continuous, fartleks	
Threshold	5–8 a side	Fartleks, skill/run circuits	
Maximal aerobic	3–4 a side	Max Aerobic courses/runs	
Maximal intervals	1–2 a side	Multidirectional runs, sprint relays	

Tec/tac training (technical and tactical training) features in the plans when physical development is not paramount, allowing you to concentrate on developing those skills. This is normally done close to competition, for athletes at all levels, as it has a low training load and ensures the athlete is fresh for competition and the tactics are fresh in their mind.

SKILL-BASED ENDURANCE SPORT SCHEDULE

Phase	Monday	Tuesday	Wednesday
Week 1: build, mainly aerobic base	Tec/tac ~20 minutes Steady ~3 × 12 minutes	Tec/tac ~20 minutes Threshold 5 × ~5 minutes Strength session 1	Rest day
Training Load Gauges			
Week 2: use all endurance methods, build volume	Tec/tac ~20 minutes Threshold 6 × 5 minutes Max intervals 2 sets of 4 × 20 seconds @ 95% max, 60 seconds rest, 2 minutes per set Strength session 1	Steady ~2 × 20 minutes Max aerobic 4 × 3½ minutes, 2 minutes rest	Rest day
Training Load Gauges			
Week 3: build volume and match exposure	Tec/tac ~20 minutes Threshold 3 × 12 minutes Max intervals 2 sets of 4 × 20 seconds @ 95% max, 45 seconds rest, 2 minutes per set Strength session 1	Tec/tac ~30 minutes Steady ~2 × 25 minutes Max aerobic 4 × 4 minutes, 2 minutes rest	Rest day
Training Load Gauges			

Thursday	Friday	Saturday	Sunday
Tec/tac ~30 minutes Steady ~4 × 10 minutes	Threshold 5 × ~5 minutes Max intervals 2 sets of 4 × 15 seconds @ 95% max, 45 seconds rest, 2 minutes per set Strength session 2	Steady ~3 × 10 minutes Max aerobic 4 × 3 minutes, 2 minutes rest	Rest day
Tec/tac ~20 minutes Threshold 6 × 6 minutes Max intervals 2 sets of 4 × 20 seconds @ 95% max, 45 seconds rest, 2 minutes per set Strength session 2	Tec/tac 60 minutes	Practice match ~half normal match	Rest day
Tec/tac ~30 minutes Threshold 6 × 7 minutes Max intervals – 4 × 50 metres, 6 × 30 metres, 8 × 15 metres × 1:4 rest* Strength session 2	Tec/tac 60 minutes	Practice match ~two-thirds normal match (split squad)	Rest day

Training bar key: ○ steady ○ threshold ○ max aerobic ● max intervals ○ mixed training

Abbreviations: ~ approximately

*However long your work time, the rest period is a ratio of this, i.e., if you work for 10 seconds a work:rest ratio of 1:4 would mean resting for 40 seconds.

SKILL-BASED ENDURANCE SPORT SCHEDULE

Phase	Monday	Tuesday	Wednesday
Week 4: **use greater volume of intense methods**	Tec/tac ~20 minutes Threshold 3 × 12 minutes Max intervals 2 sets of 4 × 20 seconds @ 95% max, 45 seconds rest, 2 minutes per set Strength session 1	Tec/tac ~30 minutes Steady ~2 × 30 minutes Max aerobic 4 × 4 minutes, 2 minutes rest	Rest day
Training Load Gauges			
Week 5: **build competition minutes and maximise volume**	Tec/tac ~30 minutes Max aerobic 3 × 2 minutes, 1 minute rest Strength session 2	Friendly match ~ 80% usual match duration**	Rest day
Training Load Gauges			
Week 6: **taper for season start**	Tec/tac ~30 minutes Threshold ~3 × 6 minutes Strength session 1	Steady ~2 × 10 minutes Max aerobic 4 × 3 minutes, 2 minutes rest	Rest day
Training Load Gauges			

Thursday	Friday	Saturday	Sunday
Tec/tac ~30 minutes Threshold 6 × 7 minutes Max intervals –4 × 50 metres, 6 × 30metres, 8 × 15 metres @ 100%, 1:3 rest* Strength session 2	Tec/tac ~60 minutes	Practice match ~75% normal match	Rest day
Tec/tac ~30 minutes Threshold 3 × 7 minutes Max intervals 4 × 40 metres, 6 × 20metres, 8 × 10m @ 100%, 1:3 rest* Strength session 1	Tec/tac ~60 minutes	Practice match ~full match	Rest day
Tec/tac ~45 minutes Max intervals 100% 2 × 40 metres, 4 × 20 metres, 6 × 10 metres @ 100%, 1:4 rest* Strength session 2	Tec/tac ~60 minutes	First competitive match	Rest day

Training bar key: ⬤ steady ⬤ threshold ⬤ max aerobic ⬤ max intervals ⬤ mixed training

Abbreviations: ~ approximately

*However long your work time, the rest period is a ratio of this, i.e., if you work for 10 seconds a work:rest ratio of 1:4 would mean resting for 40 seconds.

**Play at least 80% of normal match duration: so for football, which is 90 minutes, play at least 72 minutes; for hockey, which is 70 minutes, play at least 56 minutes.

Strength Training

The principal aim of this strength plan is to enhance speed, duel strength, endurance efficiency and robustness to injury. The plan involves two sessions per week with equipment typically found in a gym. Two strength sessions per week have been shown to be sufficient in developing strength qualities in high-level athletes; however, some sports, such as rugby, rely more on the strength and size of players, so if this applies to your sport you might want to perform more sessions with greater emphasis on muscle size training.

Strength max provides the max

Most of the strength exercises are performed in the Strength Max range (3–5 sets of 1–6 repetitions) because it provides so many benefits. If you run as part of your sport, you want to be as strong, but as lean, as possible, because you need to move your body against the force of gravity. Greater maximum strength improves our acceleration, and a high strength-to-bodyweight ratio means that we use less energy for a given action, so our endurance improves. Good maximum strength also means that you can be strong in duels that happen frequently in team sports, and you will be less likely to get injured from the impact of running. Power training, such as jumps, throws and Olympic lifts, are also important because high-power actions are typically the key moments in team sports, such as taking on your opponents to score; however, they do not form a huge part of this programme, as aspects such as sprints and jumps are performed regularly as part of the field training.

Optimise session flow

Both programmes are whole-body based and commence with power exercises or leg-strength exercises to take advantage of being fresh, and the production of growth hormones from large-muscle-mass exercises. The first session has a greater focus on leg-strength development and is used further away from competition so as to overcome greater leg fatigue. The leg-strength exercises have a bias towards training the posterior of the body to help prevent hamstring injuries, which are common in field sports. The second session is more focused on power and injury prevention and has a lighter leg load so that it can be used closer to practice competition. Exercises are performed back-to-back in pairs, indicated by the number (such as 1a and 1b), using different muscle groups in order to be time efficient.

Be specific

The programmes principally use exercises that have similar movements or recruitment patterns to that seen in the sport. Using free-weight exercises, such as squats and cable exercises, is a good way to achieve this. During most sporting actions, our core muscles act as a stable anchor on the pelvis and spine so that we can move our arms and legs effectively or hold off an opponent. Therefore, the chosen core exercises involve a stable core area and are integrated into many of the upper-body exercises by performing standing cable exercises or standing on one leg.

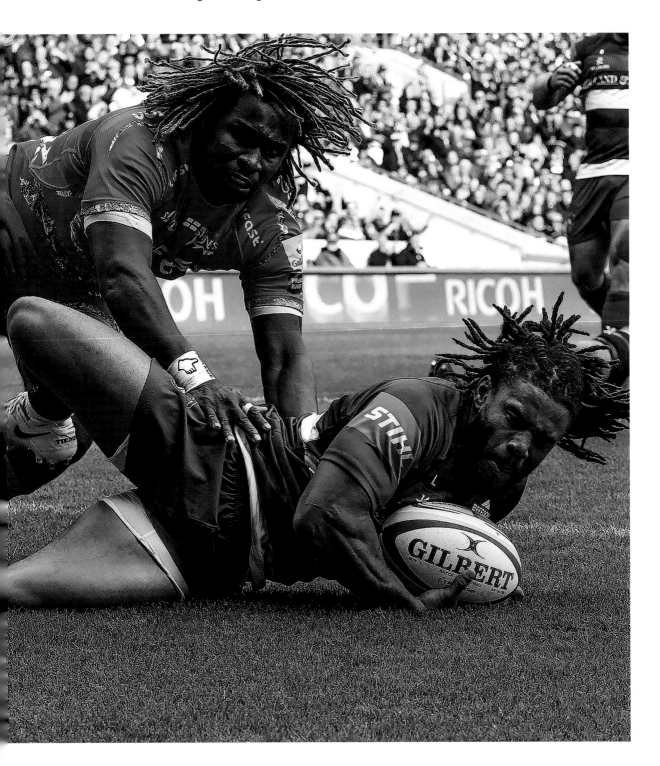

SESSION 1

LEG, UPPER BODY AND CORE; STRENGTH-SIZE PROGRESS TO MAXIMAL STRENGTH

1a Back squat	Coaching cues	Week	Structure
	Stand with the bar on your upper back. Keeping heels down, back straight and knees aligned, squat down, moving the hips back as if sitting. Aim for thighs to be parallel to ground and return to the start position.	1	3 × 8
		2	3 × 8
		3	3 × 6
		4	3 × 6
		5	6-5-4-4*
		6	6-5-4-3*

1b Bench	Coaching cues	Week	Structure
	Keeping your back flat on the bench, arms shoulder-width apart, lower the barbell to your chest, pause, then push back to start position.	1	3 × 8
		2	3 × 8
		3	3 × 6
		4	3 × 6
		5	6-5-4-4*
		6	6-5-4-3*

2a Romanian deadlift	Coaching cues	Week	Structure
	Stand with barbell, knees slightly bent. Move hips backwards and lower barbell down close to the body, keeping back straight. Once you feel the hamstrings stretched, reverse the movement, pushing the hips through.	1	3 × 8
		2	3 × 8
		3	3 × 6
		4	3 × 6
		5	6-5-4-4*
		6	6-5-4-4*

2b Pull-up	Coaching cues	Week	Structure
	Begin hanging from the bar, arms shoulder-width apart. Pull yourself up to the bar, once the chin clears the bar, lower back to full extension.	1	3 × TF with BW
		2	3 × TF with BW
		3	3 × TF with 5kg
		4	3 × TF with 5kg
		5	3 × TF with 10kg
		6	3 × TF with 10kg

3a Lunge cable pull	Coaching cues	Week	Structure
	Get into lunge position and grab the cable with the opposite hand to the forward-lunge leg. Pull the cable towards your hip and return to the start position.	1	3 × 10
		2	3 × 10
		3	3 × 8
		4	3 × 8
		5	3 × 6
		6	3 × 6

3b Swiss ball roll out	Coaching cues	Week	Structure
	Place full forearm on the Swiss ball so that your upper arm is perpendicular to your body. Keeping a straight line through the body, move your arm up, pushing the ball away from your body until your back begins to arch, then pull it back to the start position.	1	3 × 10
		2	3 × 10
		3	3 × 10
		4	3 × 12
		5	3 × 12
		6	3 × 12

NOTE: *Perform the same number of exercises as pairs to reduce rest (about 1 minute between each)*

TF = to fatigue | BW = bodyweight

* see page 234 for explanation of sequence of numbers used for reps

SESSION 2

LEG POWER AND PROTECTION, UPPER AND CORE SIZE AND MAX STRENGTH

1a Single leg box jump	Coaching cues	Week	Structure
	Stand on one leg, hop maximally onto an elevated surface. Step down gently before repeating.	1	2 × 4 each leg
		2	2 × 4 each leg
		3	2 × 5 each leg
		4	2 × 5 each leg
		5	3 × 4 each leg
		6	3 × 4 each leg

1b Cable press	Coaching cues	Week	Structure
	Hold cable slightly below shoulder height and wider than the chest. Press forward and in until the arms are straight, then return to the start position .	1	3 × 10
		2	3 × 10
		3	3 × 8
		4	3 × 8
		5	3 × 6
		6	3 × 6

2a Rear foot elevated squats	Coaching cues	Week	Structure
	Hold dumbbells and place one leg on an elevated surface behind you, positioning the front foot so that the shin is roughly vertical. With weight on front foot, lower yourself until the front thigh is parallel with the ground, push through the heels to return to start position.	1	3 × 8 each leg
		2	3 × 8 each leg
		3	3 × 6 each leg
		4	3 × 6 each leg
		5	6–5-4 each leg*
		6	6-5-4 each leg*

2b Seated cable pull	Coaching cues	Week	Structure
	Sit holding cable and feet against a secure surface. Slightly bent at the knee, with back straight, chest out, pull the cable towards your belly and return to the start position	1	3 × 8 each arm
		2	3 × 8 each arm
		3	3 × 6 each arm
		4	3 × 6 each arm
		5	6-5-4*
		6	6–5–4*

3a Nordics	Coaching cues	Week	Structure
	Secure your heels using a partner, bar or weight. Keeping the body straight, lower your body under control by letting the knees straighten until you cannot control movements. Use your hands to return to start position.	1	3 × 4
		2	3 × 4
		3	3 × 6
		4	3 × 6
		5	3 × 8
		6	3 × 8

3b One arm and leg press	Coaching cues	Week	Structure
	Stand on one leg, with opposite arm holding a dumbbell at shoulder height, push the dumbbell up above your head until fully extended, then return to start position.	1	3 × 10 each arm
		2	3 × 10 each arm
		3	3 × 8 each arm
		4	3 × 8 each arm
		5	3 × 6 each arm
		6	3 × 6 each arm

NOTE: *Perform the same number of exercises as pairs to reduce rest (about 1–2 minutes between each)*

* see page 234 for explanation of sequence of numbers used for reps

Meal plan: skill-based endurance sport

The meal plan below shows a sample one-week plan. The training structure is similar for all weeks, so the plan provides a suitable meal structure for the whole programme. The key principle is that the Fuel foods and meals are varied in line with training activity and competition schedules, ensuring you have sufficient energy to support the high training loads. See page 280 for more information.

	Monday	Tuesday	Wednesday
	Training Morning training Training load Moderate Rationale Focus on Fuel to support training; balanced otherwise	Training Morning training, afternoon strength Training load Hard Rationale Focus on Fuel for training and add Lean Muscle post strength exercises	Training Rest day Training load n/a Rationale Health and Lean Muscle take priority but some Fuel restoration
Breakfast	Apple and Cinnamon Pancakes (page 29)	Zesty Quinoa Porridge (page 34)	Courgette Pancakes (page 52)
Morning snack	No snack	No snack	No snack
Lunch	Chickpea Chaat (page 89)	Tortilla Pizza and Cajun Street Rice (pages 73 and 140)	Prawn and Asparagus Stir-Fry (page 71)
Afternoon snack	Sugar-free granola	Protein Frappuccino (page 187)	Cracker and cottage cheese
Dinner	Spicy Prawns and Quinoa (page 97)	Roasted Vegetable Lasagne (page 92)	Salmon, Tomato and Asparagus Bake (page 98)
Evening snack	Wholemeal toast and almond butter	Almond Cobbler (page 157)	No snack

Thursday	Friday	Saturday	Sunday
Training Morning training, afternoon strength Training load Moderate Rationale Balanced as training load is moderate; Lean Muscle post strength exercises	Training Morning training Training load Light Rationale Fuel takes priority for upcoming match	Training Afternoon match Training load Very hard Rationale Focus on Fuel prior to match; Fuel and Lean Muscle post match for recovery	Training Rest day Training load n/a Rationale Health and Lean Muscle take priority, but some Fuel for restoration
Scrambled eggs and wholemeal toast	Overnight Oats (see Overnight Oats Meal Builder, page 56)	Beetroot and Mixed Berry Smoothie and Almond and Banana Pancakes (pages 185 and 39)	Kiwi and Banana Parfait (page 33)
No snack	No snack	Carrot Cake Balls (page 164)	No snack
Peanut Butter Tempeh with Stir-Fry Noodles (page 95)	Mediterranean Wrap and Salt and Pepper Sweet Potato Chips (pages 76 and 146)	Pre-match meal: flaked salmon and pasta with sauce and a banana or rice pudding pot	Tuscan Bean Soup (page 62) with bread
Whey protein shake with milk (see Smoothie Builder, page 192)	Berries and Greek yogurt	Post-match: milk shake (see Smoothie Builder, page 192) and chicken salad wrap (see Wrap and Sandwich Builder, page 82)	Beef jerky
Turkey Burger, Spiced Bulgar Wheat (pages 118 and 135) and mixed veg	Chinese Beef Noodles (page 123)	Chicken and Mushroom Risotto (page 113)	Steak, roast asparagus and new potatoes
Mocha Parfait (page 30)	Poached egg on toast	Sugar-free granola	No snack

Pre-season = hard training = lots of fuelling

Pre-season typically involves the highest volume of training for field-sport athletes, with regular hard-field training, strength training and practice competitions. Fuel is a dominant feature to support training and match performance. Starting a match with high carb stores has been shown to improve total and high-intensity distance covered, in addition to skill maintenance, decision making and injury prevention. This is why fuel intake the day before a match remains high, despite training demands being quite low. The plan involves three main meals and two snacks on training days to support the high calorie and fuel requirements.

Lean Muscle foods also feature frequently and are emphasised after hard training, strength training and competition to promote muscular recovery and development. Health is maximised at all opportunities and emphasised on rest days.

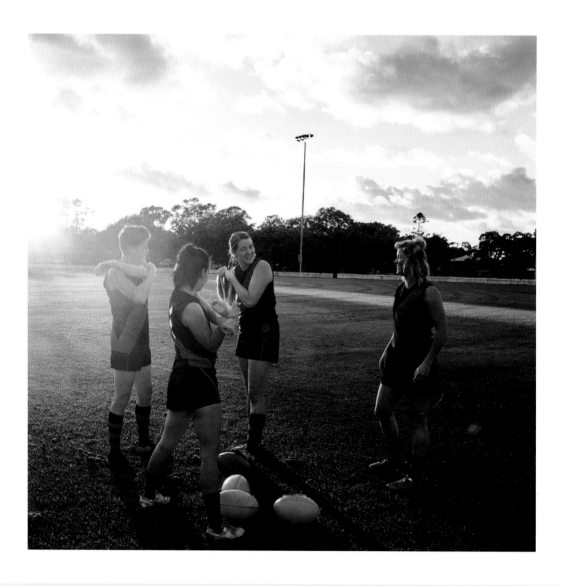

Index

Acknowledgements

As with everything good in my life, I'd like to acknowledge the role of my incredible wife, Emma, and kids, Isabelle and James – thank you for your constant support and the joy you bring every day.

I'm grateful to the vast array of experts who helped me develop the Colour-Fit methodology, especially in the early days, with nutritionist Mark Hearris and chef Loren Cole both being integral. I'm particularly grateful to my wingman Luke Hemmings, whose kindness and work ethic know no bounds. I'm indebted to those at hero, and especially Joe Gaunt, for believing in and developing Colour-Fit into the navigator app, which allowed the method to grow and help people all around the world.

This book would not exist without the unwavering belief of my literary agent Jonathan Conway – thank you. I'd also like to thank the brilliant editorial team at Piatkus – Zoe Bohm, Jillian Stewart and Jillian Young – for their amazing guidance and eye for detail, and the designer, Sian Rance, for bringing the book to life.

Finally, I'd like to thank the thousands of athletes I've had the good fortune to have worked with, especially the challenging ones who created the spark for Colour-Fit. Long may you be a pain in my rear.